HIDDEN CASH FLOW IN MEDICAL PRACTICES

A Comprehensive Guide

Contents

Introduction 1

Chapter 1: Mastering Deferred Income 5

Chapter 2: The Power of Prepaid Services 9

Chapter 3: Mastering the Power of Capitation Payments 15

Chapter 4: Mastering the Management of Uncollected
      Co-Pays and Deductibles 19

Chapter 5: Mastering Discounts and Write-Offs 25

Chapter 6: Mastering the Maze of Insurance Delays 29

Chapter 7: Mastering Rebates and Incentives from Suppliers 35

Chapter 8: Mastering Investment Income 41

Chapter 9: Mastering Grants and Donations for
      Financial Growth 47

Chapter 10: Mastering the Advantages of Leasing Equipment ... 53

Chapter 11: Mastering Deferred Tax Liabilities for
      Financial Success 57

Chapter 12: Mastering Partnership Distributions for
      Financial Success 61

Chapter 13: Mastering Expense Reimbursements for
      Financial Efficiency 67

Chapter 14: Mastering the Management of Loan Proceeds 73

Chapter 15: Mastering Contributions to Employee Benefit Plans... 77

Chapter 16: Mastering Income from Legal Settlements................ 81

Chapter 17: Mastering Non-Operating Income Sources for Financial Growth 85

Chapter 18: Mastering Barter Transactions for Financial Success.. 91

Chapter 19: Mastering Income from Research Activities 95

Chapter 20: Mastering Vendor Financing Arrangements for Financial Flexibility 101

Chapter 21: Mastering Delayed Recognition of Credit Card Payments.. 107

Chapter 22: Mastering Deferred Revenue from Subscription Services.. 111

Chapter 23: Mastering Advance Payments for Future Services 117

Chapter 24: Mastering Income from Joint Ventures 121

Chapter 25: Mastering Special Discounts from Bulk Purchases 127

Conclusion: Unleashing Hidden Cash Flow in Your Medical Practice 131

Introduction

In the world of medical practices, where every decision can mean the difference between thriving and merely surviving, mastering the art of financial management is not just an option—it's a necessity. Picture this: your practice is like a high-performance sports car. It looks great, runs well, and takes you where you need to go. But what if I told you that under the hood, there are hidden gears and turbochargers that could skyrocket your performance to levels you never imagined? That's exactly what managing your cash flow effectively can do for your medical practice.

Most doctors and medical professionals I talk to are laser-focused on patient care. And rightly so! Delivering top-notch care is why you got into this field. But here's the kicker: while you're busy saving lives and enhancing patient experiences, a significant chunk of your potential income is slipping through the cracks. We're talking about $50,000 or more in hidden cash flow every single month. Let that sink in for a moment. That's over $600,000 a year without seeing a single new patient!

Now, imagine what your practice could do with that kind of extra revenue. State-of-the-art equipment, expanding your team, upgrading your facilities, or even opening a new location. The possibilities are endless. And it all starts with uncovering and recapturing that hidden cash flow.

This book is your roadmap to financial empowerment in your medical practice. We're not talking about shady shortcuts or dubious practices. Everything here is above board, legal, and used by the savviest practices across the country. I've teamed up with top CPAs and attorneys nationwide to bring you the most effective strategies for uncovering hidden cash flows and maximizing your revenue potential.

Let me paint a picture for you. Dr. Smith runs a bustling orthopedic clinic in the heart of the city. He's got a loyal patient base, a skilled team, and an impressive clinic. But despite his success, he felt like there was something more he could be doing to improve his bottom line. That's when he discovered the principles in this book. By applying these strategies, Dr. Smith identified over $75,000 in hidden cash flow each month. Within a year, he had overhauled his clinic, invested in cutting-edge technology, and even started a new fellowship program. His practice didn't just grow — it exploded.

How did Dr. Dansey do it? By understanding and implementing the legal methods of managing hidden cash flow that we'll explore in this book. He learned to leverage deferred income, optimize prepaid services, and utilize various financial tools to keep his cash flow steady and strong.

Here's the deal: deferred income, prepaid services, capitation payments, uncollected co-pays, and insurance delays — these are just a few of the areas where money can get tied up. When you know how to manage these effectively, you transform potential income into actual revenue. And that's just the beginning. We'll dive into how to handle rebates, investment income, grants, donations, and even non-operating income sources like selling old equipment or property.

Think about the impact on your cash flow when you start accounting for these hidden revenues. Imagine the peace of mind knowing that you're maximizing every dollar that comes into your practice. This book will show you how to do just that. We'll break down complex concepts into easy-to-understand strategies that you can implement immediately.

We're talking about practical, actionable steps. You'll learn how to automate your billing systems, conduct regular financial reviews, and forecast cash flow with precision. You'll discover the power of clear contract terms and open communication with clients. And you'll see how compliance with accounting standards not only keeps you in the clear legally but also builds trust with your patients, employees, and investors.

One of the biggest game-changers is learning how to recognize revenue correctly over time. Take those orthodontic treatment plans we'll discuss—recording deferred income accurately can revolutionize your financial statements. It aligns your revenue with the services provided, giving you a true picture of your financial health and enabling better decision-making.

So, are you ready to transform your practice? Are you ready to uncover the hidden cash flow that's waiting to be claimed? This book is your key to unlocking that potential. With the expertise of top CPAs and attorneys backing you, you'll be equipped to take your practice to new heights.

This book offers educational content designed to enhance your understanding of cash flow management within medical practices. This content is intended for informational purposes only and should not be construed as professional financial, accounting, or legal advice. For specific guidance tailored to your unique situation, please consult with licensed professionals in the fields of finance, accounting, or law. Additionally, please note that all case studies included in this material were researched using publicly available sources and are provided for illustrative purposes only.

To get started, scan the QR code below to find out just how much hidden cash flow you're giving away every month. Don't let another dollar slip through your fingers. It's time to take control, maximize your revenue, and elevate your practice to the next level. Welcome to the journey of discovering hidden cash flow in your medical practice. Let's get started!

CHAPTER 1:

Mastering Deferred Income

Alright, let's talk about one of the most critical and often misunderstood aspects of financial management in a medical practice: deferred income. Picture this: you've got a steady stream of patients, your services are top-notch, but there's a chunk of revenue that isn't showing up in your bank account just yet. That, my friends, is deferred income—earnings that you've generated but haven't yet pocketed. Understanding and mastering deferred income can make a world of difference in your cash flow management and overall financial health. So, let's dive deep and turn this concept into a powerful tool for your practice.

Deferred income is like a financial time bomb—in a good way. It's revenue that you've earned by providing services, but you won't actually receive the cash until later. This situation is typical in medical practices where long-term treatment plans are common. For instance, let's say you're running an orthodontic practice. A patient signs up for a two-year treatment plan costing $6,000. You can't recognize all that money upfront because the services will be provided over two years. Instead, you recognize the income gradually as the treatment progresses.

Now, why is this important? Because it impacts how you view your financial health and manage your cash flow. Deferred income ensures that your financial statements reflect the true state of your business, matching revenue with the period in which it's earned.

Let's break down the accounting side of things. When you receive payment for a long-term service plan, it initially goes on your balance sheet as a liability under deferred revenue. This isn't money you've earned yet; it's a promise to provide services in the future. For our orthodontic example, when you get that $6,000 upfront, you record it as deferred revenue. As each month of treatment goes by, you recognize a portion of that revenue. If the treatment plan is spread evenly over 24 months, you'll recognize $250 per month as income. This approach ensures your revenue recognition aligns with the service delivery, keeping your financial records accurate and transparent.

Managing deferred income requires strategic thinking and meticulous accounting. You need to track these deferred revenues accurately and update your books regularly to reflect the income as it's earned. Implementing automated billing and accounting systems can make this process seamless. These systems help track deferred income and ensure timely revenue recognition, reducing manual errors and administrative burdens.

Consider Dr. Anderson, who runs a successful dermatology practice offering a year-long skincare program. Patients pay $1,200 upfront, and the program includes monthly treatments and products. Initially, Dr. Anderson struggled with managing this deferred income manually, which led to financial discrepancies and confusion. After implementing an automated billing system, she could track deferred revenue accurately. Each month, $100 was recognized as income, providing a clear picture of her monthly revenue. This clarity allowed Dr. Anderson to manage her cash flow better, invest in new equipment, and even expand her practice.

Another strategy is maintaining a separate deferred revenue account to avoid mixing it with your operational income. This segregation helps in better financial planning and ensures you have a clear view of your actual earnings versus future commitments. Regularly reviewing and reconciling your deferred income accounts is crucial to avoid discrepancies and ensure accuracy.

Let's look at a real-world example of effective deferred income management. Dr. Martinez runs a pediatric clinic offering annual wellness plans for $1,000. Initially, he recorded the entire amount as revenue upfront, which distorted his financial statements and led to cash flow issues. After consulting with a financial advisor, Dr. Martinez started recording the $1,000 as deferred revenue and recognized $83.33 each month. This change provided a more accurate financial picture, allowing him to plan better for future expenses and investments. As a result, his clinic's financial health improved, and he could expand his services without financial strain.

Deferred income isn't just about managing numbers; it's about strategic financial planning. By understanding and effectively managing deferred income, you can ensure a stable cash flow, accurate financial statements, and a solid foundation for growth. This approach transforms deferred income from a potential financial headache into a strategic advantage, allowing you to focus on what you do best: providing excellent patient care.

In conclusion, mastering deferred income is essential for any medical practice looking to maintain financial health and drive growth. By accurately accounting for and strategically managing deferred income, you can ensure your financial statements reflect your true earnings and position your practice for long-term success. So, embrace the power of deferred income, implement robust accounting practices, and watch your practice thrive. This isn't just about managing revenue — it's about leveraging it to build a stronger, more prosperous practice. Let's turn those deferred dollars into tangible growth and stability, and take your practice to the next level!

CHAPTER 2:

The Power of Prepaid Services

Alright, let's get real about something that can transform your medical practice's financial game: prepaid services. Imagine a world where cash flow issues are a thing of the past, where you have money in the bank before you even provide a service. Sounds like a dream, right? Well, that's the power of prepaid services. When managed correctly, prepaid services can be a game-changer, providing financial stability and flexibility. So, let's dive deep into how you can leverage prepaid services to enhance your cash flow while keeping everything transparent and compliant.

Prepaid services are exactly what they sound like: payments you receive upfront for services you will deliver in the future. This isn't just about getting paid early; it's about creating a financial cushion that allows you to invest, expand, and innovate without constantly worrying about immediate revenue. Think of it as securing your financial future one payment at a time. For medical practices, this can take various forms, from annual wellness plans to prepaid packages for elective procedures.

Take Dr. Stevens, a successful orthodontist. He offers a prepaid treatment plan for braces, which spans two years and costs $5,000. Patients pay the full amount upfront, securing their treatment and giving Dr. Stevens a significant cash influx. This setup not only assures patients that they are committed to a comprehensive treatment plan but also provides Dr. Stevens with the financial flexibility to invest in cutting-edge equipment and hire additional staff without the constant stress of cash flow management.

But here's the kicker: managing these prepaid services effectively requires meticulous accounting and strategic planning. When you receive that $5,000 upfront, it doesn't go straight into your revenue. Instead, it's recorded as a liability on your balance sheet under deferred revenue. Why? Because you haven't earned it yet. You'll earn it gradually as you provide the service over the two years. Each month, as Dr. Stevens adjusts those braces, a portion of that prepaid amount gets recognized as revenue. This way, your financial statements accurately reflect your earnings and obligations, ensuring transparency and compliance.

Let's break it down with an example. Suppose Dr. Stevens decides to recognize $208.33 each month as revenue over the 24 months of treatment. In the first month, he records the full $5,000 as deferred revenue. Then, each month, he reduces this liability and recognizes the $208.33 as income. This approach not only aligns with accounting standards but also provides a clear financial picture, showing both your obligations and your earned income.

Now, let's talk about the benefits and challenges of prepaid services. The most obvious benefit is improved cash flow. With money in the bank before services are rendered, you have the liquidity to cover operational costs, invest in growth opportunities, and navigate financial uncertainties with ease. This upfront cash can be a lifesaver during slow periods, ensuring you maintain a steady operation without dipping into reserves or taking on debt.

Another significant advantage is patient commitment. When patients prepay for services, they're more likely to follow through with treatments, attend appointments, and adhere to prescribed care plans. This commitment not only improves patient outcomes but also enhances the efficiency of your practice by reducing no-shows and cancellations. Patients are more invested, quite literally, in their healthcare journey, fostering a stronger patient-provider relationship.

However, managing prepaid services isn't without its challenges. One of the primary challenges is ensuring accurate and transparent accounting. Mismanaging deferred revenue can lead to financial discrepancies and compliance issues, potentially damaging your reputation and financial health. This is where implementing a robust accounting system becomes crucial. Automated billing and accounting software can track deferred revenue, ensure timely recognition of income, and maintain detailed records for audits and financial reviews.

Consider Dr. Patel, who runs a multi-specialty clinic offering a variety of prepaid wellness packages. Initially, he struggled with manual tracking, leading to financial discrepancies and patient dissatisfaction. After switching to an automated system, Dr. Patel not only streamlined the management of prepaid services but also improved patient satisfaction. The system tracked each payment, scheduled revenue recognition, and provided detailed reports, allowing Dr. Patel to focus on expanding his services rather than worrying about financial management.

Transparency is another critical aspect. Clear communication with patients about the terms and benefits of prepaid services is essential. Patients need to understand what they're paying for, how the payments are structured, and what happens if they need to cancel or reschedule. Providing detailed information upfront builds trust and ensures patients are fully aware of their commitments.

Take the example of Dr. Lee, who runs a pediatric practice. She introduced a prepaid annual wellness plan, providing comprehensive care for children at a discounted rate. By clearly communicating the benefits and terms, including detailed brochures and personal consultations, Dr. Lee built a strong foundation of trust with her patients. This transparency not only boosted enrollments in the wellness plan but also enhanced overall patient satisfaction and retention.

Now, let's look at a real-world case study to see these concepts in action. Dr. Ramirez, an aesthetic surgeon, decided to offer prepaid packages for elective cosmetic procedures. These packages, priced at $10,000, covered consultations, surgeries, and post-operative care. Dr. Ramirez used an automated system to manage the deferred revenue, recognizing income as each stage of the treatment was completed. This approach provided him with a significant upfront cash flow, allowing him to invest in advanced surgical tools and a state-of-the-art clinic.

The results were astounding. Dr. Ramirez's clinic saw a 40% increase in patient enrollment for prepaid packages within the first year. The improved cash flow enabled him to expand his team and enhance patient care, further boosting his clinic's reputation and attracting even more patients. The transparency and structured payment plan built trust with his patients, ensuring they fully understood the value and benefits of their investment.

In conclusion, prepaid services, when managed effectively, can revolutionize your medical practice's financial health. By understanding the nuances of deferred revenue, implementing robust accounting practices, and maintaining transparency with your patients, you can harness the power of prepaid services to enhance cash flow, improve patient commitment, and drive growth. So, embrace the potential of prepaid services, invest in the right systems, and watch your practice thrive. Let's turn those upfront payments into a solid foundation for success and take your practice to new heights!

CHAPTER 3:

Mastering the Power of Capitation Payments

Let's dive into a financial strategy that can bring stability and predictability to your medical practice's revenue: capitation payments. Imagine a scenario where you receive a steady, predictable income each month, regardless of how many patients walk through your doors. Sounds too good to be true? It's not. Capitation payments, when understood and managed correctly, can transform the way you operate, providing financial stability and enhancing your cash flow.

Capitation payments are a financial model where you get paid a set amount per patient, per period, rather than per service rendered. This means that for every patient enrolled under your care, you receive a fixed monthly payment. Whether they visit your practice once or ten times, the payment remains the same. This model shifts the focus from quantity to quality of care, incentivizing you to keep patients healthy and reduce unnecessary visits.

To truly grasp how capitation payments work, let's consider Dr. Smith, who runs a busy family practice. He signs a contract with an insurance provider that agrees to pay him $30 per month for each enrolled patient. With 1,000 patients, Dr. Smith knows he'll receive $30,000 every month, regardless of the number of services provided. This predictable income stream allows Dr.

Smith to plan better, invest in his practice, and focus on preventive care, knowing his revenue is steady.

The benefits of capitation payments are significant. First and foremost, they provide predictable revenue. Unlike fee-for-service models, where income can fluctuate wildly based on patient visits and procedures, capitation payments ensure a steady cash flow. This stability allows for better financial planning and reduces the stress associated with revenue uncertainty. Dr. Smith, for example, can confidently budget for staff salaries, rent, and other overhead costs, knowing that his income is secure.

Another major benefit is the emphasis on preventive care. Since the payment is fixed, the incentive shifts from providing more services to keeping patients healthier, thereby reducing the need for frequent visits. This not only improves patient outcomes but also enhances the efficiency of your practice. Dr. Smith notices that by focusing on preventive measures like regular check-ups, health education, and early intervention, his patients stay healthier, and his practice runs more smoothly.

However, capitation payments also come with challenges. One significant drawback is the financial risk associated with high-cost patients. If several patients require extensive care, the fixed payment might not cover the costs, potentially straining your practice's finances. This model requires a careful balance of patient care and cost management. Dr. Smith must ensure that while he promotes preventive care, he also manages high-cost cases efficiently to maintain financial viability.

Accounting for capitation payments requires a shift in how you manage your books. Since the payments are received monthly, they need to be recorded as revenue for that period, ensuring your financial statements reflect the steady income. This method provides a clear picture of your financial health and helps in long-term planning. Dr. Smith's accountant records the $30,000 monthly payment as revenue, providing a stable financial overview that supports strategic decision-making.

Now, let's look at real-world applications to see how capitation payments can be successfully implemented. Dr. Lee runs a pediatric clinic and transitioned to a capitation model. She signed contracts with multiple insurance providers, ensuring a broad patient base. With 1,500 enrolled patients and an average capitation payment of $25 per patient per month, Dr. Lee receives $37,500 monthly. This steady income allows her to invest in new medical equipment, hire additional staff, and expand her clinic's services.

Dr. Lee's focus on preventive care has significantly improved patient outcomes. She implements regular wellness check-ups, immunization programs, and health education workshops. The result? Healthier children, fewer emergency visits, and a more efficient practice. Financially, the predictable revenue stream has allowed her to plan for future expansions and ensure her clinic's long-term stability.

On the flip side, consider Dr. Green, who faced challenges with the capitation model. Running a practice with many high-cost elderly patients, he initially struggled to balance the fixed income with the high cost of care. However, by implementing a comprehensive care management program, focusing on preventive measures, and closely monitoring patient health, Dr. Green managed to reduce overall healthcare costs and improve patient outcomes. This approach balanced the financial risks and benefits, demonstrating that with the right strategies, capitation payments can be effectively managed.

In conclusion, capitation payments offer a powerful model for financial stability and improved patient care in medical practices. By shifting the focus from the volume of services to the quality of care, they provide a predictable income stream that supports better financial planning and patient outcomes. Understanding the intricacies of capitation payments, managing the associated risks, and implementing effective preventive care strategies are key to leveraging this model successfully. Just like Dr. Smith and Dr. Lee, you can transform your practice, ensuring stability, growth, and enhanced patient care through the power of capitation payments. Let's embrace this model, manage it wisely, and watch your practice thrive like never before.

CHAPTER 4:

Mastering the Management of Uncollected Co-Pays and Deductibles

Alright, let's dive into one of the most persistent challenges facing medical practices today: managing uncollected co-pays and deductibles. These uncollected amounts can create hidden receivables that silently erode your practice's cash flow, causing significant financial stress and operational inefficiencies. But with the right strategies, you can turn this around, ensuring that every dollar earned makes its way into your bank account. Let's break down the challenges, implement effective collection strategies, and integrate robust accounting practices to master the management of uncollected co-pays and deductibles.

Uncollected co-pays and deductibles are like leaks in a bucket. No matter how much water you pour in, it will never fill up if you don't fix the holes. For medical practices, these uncollected amounts arise from patients failing to pay their portion of the healthcare costs, either due to forgetfulness, financial difficulties, or confusion about their insurance coverage. This situation is further complicated by the administrative burden of tracking and collecting these payments. The result? Hidden receivables that obscure your true financial position and strain your cash flow.

Consider Dr. Thompson, who runs a busy orthopedic clinic. Despite having a steady stream of patients, he noticed a troubling pattern: a growing amount of uncollected co-pays and deductibles. These hidden receivables were affecting his cash flow, making it difficult to cover operational expenses and invest in new equipment. Dr. Thompson realized that to maintain financial health, he needed a comprehensive strategy to manage these uncollected amounts.

The first step in addressing this issue is understanding the root causes. One major challenge is patient non-compliance. Some patients simply forget or neglect to pay their co-pays and deductibles, either due to misunderstanding their insurance coverage or financial difficulties. Additionally, the complexity of different insurance plans can confuse both patients and staff, leading to missed or delayed collections. Administrative oversights, such as inadequate billing systems and processes, further exacerbate the problem.

Dr. Thompson began by implementing a clear, proactive communication strategy. He ensured that patients understood their financial responsibilities upfront, providing detailed explanations of co-pays and deductibles during their initial visits. His team also sent reminders about upcoming payments, using both automated systems and personal follow-ups. This transparency helped to reduce confusion and set clear expectations, making patients more likely to comply with payment requests.

Next, Dr. Thompson revamped his billing process. He invested in an advanced practice management system that automated billing and tracked outstanding co-pays and deductibles. This system generated timely reminders for both patients and staff, ensuring that no payment was overlooked. By integrating this technology, Dr. Thompson's clinic reduced administrative burdens and improved the accuracy of their billing processes.

Effective collection strategies were also crucial. Dr. Thompson introduced a pre-visit collection policy, where patients were reminded of their financial obligations during appointment scheduling and encouraged to settle co-pays and deductibles before their visits. This approach not only improved collection rates but also reduced the administrative burden on his staff.

To handle uncollected amounts, Dr. Thompson established a structured follow-up system. His team conducted regular follow-up calls and sent emails to remind patients of their outstanding balances. They also offered multiple payment options, including online payments, to make the process as convenient as possible for patients. This consistent follow-up ensured that uncollected amounts did not linger on the books for long periods.

Accurate accounting practices played a pivotal role in managing these uncollected amounts. Dr. Thompson's accountant maintained detailed records of all patient transactions, including co-pays and deductibles. Uncollected amounts were tracked meticulously, and regular reviews were conducted to identify any discrepancies. This proactive approach helped in catching and resolving issues early, ensuring that the financial statements reflected the true financial health of the practice.

By integrating these strategies, Dr. Thompson transformed the financial management of his clinic. Improved cash flow allowed him to cover operational expenses more comfortably and invest in new technologies and services. His staff, no longer burdened by inefficient billing processes, could focus on providing excellent patient care. Patients, informed and engaged in their financial responsibilities, were more likely to comply with payment requests, further stabilizing the clinic's cash flow.

Another example is Dr. Lee, who runs a pediatric practice. She faced similar challenges with uncollected co-pays and deductibles, impacting her ability to manage expenses and plan for growth. Dr. Lee introduced a robust financial policy, clearly outlining payment expectations during patient registration. She also trained her staff to handle billing inquiries effectively, ensuring that they could provide accurate information and support to patients.

Dr. Lee's practice adopted an automated billing system that integrated with their electronic health records. This system streamlined the billing process, automatically generating invoices and reminders for outstanding payments. By reducing manual errors and administrative delays, Dr. Lee's practice saw a significant improvement in collection rates.

To further enhance financial management, Dr. Lee's accountant conducted regular audits of the billing and collection processes. These audits helped identify patterns of uncollected amounts and areas for improvement. The practice also established a reserve fund to cover potential bad debts, ensuring financial stability even when some payments remained uncollected.

Through these efforts, Dr. Lee's practice achieved a more stable cash flow and could invest in new services and patient care initiatives. The transparent and efficient handling of co-pays and deductibles improved patient satisfaction and trust, fostering a positive relationship with the community.

In conclusion, managing uncollected co-pays and deductibles is essential for maintaining the financial health of your medical practice. By understanding the challenges, implementing effective collection strategies, and maintaining accurate accounting practices, you can ensure that hidden receivables do not negatively impact your cash flow. Take control of your collections, streamline your processes, and watch your practice thrive. It's time to turn those hidden receivables into real revenue and elevate your practice to new heights. Let's make every dollar count and drive your practice toward unparalleled success!

CHAPTER 5:

Mastering Discounts and Write-Offs

Alright, let's get into the nitty-gritty of leveraging discounts and write-offs. These financial maneuvers can be powerful tools for managing patient relations and maintaining cash flow, but if not handled correctly, they can obscure the true revenue potential of your medical practice. The key is to manage them strategically, ensuring financial clarity while using them to your advantage. Let's dive deep into understanding the types of discounts and write-offs, how to account for them, and their impact on your financial statements.

First, let's define what we're talking about here. Discounts are reductions in the amount a patient owes, usually offered as an incentive for early payment, bulk services, or loyalty. Write-offs, on the other hand, are amounts that you decide to no longer pursue, often due to the realization that the debt is uncollectible. Both of these tools can help improve patient satisfaction and cash flow management, but they need to be carefully tracked to avoid financial misstatements.

Consider Dr. Thompson, who runs a thriving orthopedic practice. He offers a 10% discount to patients who pay their bills within 15 days. This discount is designed to encourage prompt payment and reduce the time his accounts receivable remain outstanding. However, every discount given also reduces the revenue reported on his financial statements, which, if not managed properly, can lead to an inaccurate picture of the practice's financial health.

To accurately account for discounts, Dr. Thompson's accountant records the full service amount as revenue and then notes the discount as a separate expense. This method maintains transparency, showing both the potential revenue and the cost of the discount. For example, if a service costs $1,000 and a 10% discount is given, the accountant records $1,000 as revenue and $100 as a discount expense. This approach ensures that financial statements reflect the true impact of discounts on revenue.

Write-offs are a different beast. They typically occur when it becomes clear that a debt cannot be collected, often due to patient bankruptcy or prolonged non-payment. Dr. Thompson might have an outstanding bill of $500 that remains unpaid for over a year despite multiple collection attempts. Realizing that continuing to pursue this debt is futile, he decides to write it off. Writing off bad debt involves removing the amount from accounts receivable and recording it as a bad debt expense. This process ensures that the financial statements no longer overstate assets and accurately reflect the practice's revenue.

The impact of discounts and write-offs on financial statements is significant. They directly reduce revenue and net income, which can affect profitability metrics and financial ratios. For instance, offering substantial discounts to attract more patients might increase cash flow in the short term but could potentially lower overall profitability if not balanced correctly. Similarly, frequent write-offs might indicate issues with patient billing or collection processes, signaling a need for tighter credit policies or better patient communication.

Dr. Thompson's practice provides a practical example of how to manage these financial tools effectively. By implementing a systematic approach to discounts, his practice offers incentives that drive timely payments without sacrificing too much revenue. For instance, the practice tracks the effectiveness of the 10% early payment discount by analyzing payment patterns and adjusting the discount rate as needed to optimize both cash flow and revenue. This data-driven approach helps maintain financial clarity while leveraging discounts to improve cash flow.

Dr. Thompson also has a robust policy for managing write-offs. His practice reviews outstanding receivables quarterly, categorizing debts based on the likelihood of collection. Debts deemed uncollectible after thorough review are written off, ensuring the accounts receivable reflect realistic expectations. This proactive approach not only maintains the integrity of financial statements but also helps the practice identify patterns or issues in billing and collection processes that might need addressing.

Another example is Dr. Lee, who runs a busy pediatric clinic. She offers a variety of discounts, including multi-child discounts for families and seasonal promotions for flu shots. Dr. Lee ensures that all discounts are recorded accurately by her accounting team, who follow a strict protocol to document each discount offered and its impact on revenue. This practice helps Dr. Lee maintain a clear picture of her clinic's financial health, enabling her to make informed decisions about future promotions and pricing strategies.

Dr. Lee also handles write-offs with a strategic mindset. Her clinic has established criteria for determining when a debt should be written off, such as after six months of non-payment and two failed collection attempts. This systematic approach ensures that write-offs are not done haphazardly but are based on consistent, transparent criteria. Dr. Lee's practice reviews write-off policies annually to ensure they align with the clinic's financial goals and regulatory requirements.

In conclusion, managing discounts and write-offs effectively requires a strategic approach and meticulous accounting practices. By understanding the types of discounts and write-offs, accurately recording them, and assessing their impact on financial statements, you can maintain financial clarity and leverage these tools to your advantage. Both Dr. Thompson and Dr. Lee's practices demonstrate that with the right strategies, discounts can enhance patient satisfaction and prompt payments, while write-offs can keep financial records accurate and reflective of true revenue potential. So, take control of your discounts and write-offs, ensure transparency in your financial reporting, and use these tools to strengthen your practice's financial health. By doing so, you'll not only improve cash flow but also build a foundation for sustainable growth and success. Let's turn these financial tools into strategic assets and elevate your practice to new heights.

CHAPTER 6:

Mastering the Maze of Insurance Delays

Alright, let's talk about a topic that every medical practice encounters but few truly master: dealing with insurance delays. These delays can create a frustrating lag between delivering a service and actually seeing the cash. It's like running a marathon and finding out you have to wait at the finish line before you can collect your prize. Understanding the causes of these delays and implementing effective strategies to manage them is crucial for maintaining a healthy cash flow and ensuring the financial stability of your practice. So, let's dive into the intricate world of insurance delays and learn how to turn this challenge into a strategic advantage.

Insurance delays are caused by a variety of factors, each one a potential stumbling block in the path to timely payment. One of the primary culprits is the complexity of the claim procedures. Insurance companies often have detailed and cumbersome processes for submitting claims, and even minor errors can lead to significant delays. Missing or incorrect information, such as incorrect patient data or coding errors, can result in claims being rejected or delayed for further verification.

Take Dr. Smith's family practice, for instance. Dr. Smith noticed that a large number of his claims were being delayed due to minor coding errors. Each error, no matter how small, required resubmission and prolonged the payment process. This realization led him to overhaul his billing process. By investing in comprehensive training for his administrative staff and implementing advanced billing software that automatically checks for common errors, Dr. Smith significantly reduced the incidence of delayed claims.

Another major cause of delays is verification issues. Insurance companies need to verify patient coverage and benefits, and any discrepancies can lead to hold-ups. Pre-authorization requirements add another layer of complexity, especially for procedures that need prior approval from the insurance company. Dr. Lee, who runs a pediatric clinic, faced frequent delays due to pre-authorization requirements. She implemented a system where her staff would verify insurance details and obtain necessary pre-authorizations before scheduling procedures. This proactive approach minimized delays and ensured smoother cash flow.

Claim denials and the subsequent appeal processes are also significant sources of delays. Insurance companies often deny claims for a variety of reasons, necessitating a lengthy appeal process. Dr. Patel, who manages a busy cardiology clinic, encountered this issue regularly. He set up a dedicated team to handle claim denials and appeals, ensuring that each case was addressed promptly and thoroughly. This team's efforts led to a higher success rate in appeals and reduced the overall delay in payments.

Administrative backlogs within insurance companies can further exacerbate the problem. High volumes of claims can lead to delays as companies struggle to process them in a timely manner. Dr. Thompson, running an orthopedic practice, found that his claims were frequently stuck in these backlogs. By establishing direct lines of communication with the insurance providers and scheduling regular follow-ups, he managed to expedite the processing of his claims.

Effective strategies for managing these delays start with streamlining the claim submission process. Investing in advanced electronic health record (EHR) systems that integrate with billing software can significantly reduce errors and speed up the submission process. Automation ensures that claims are submitted promptly and accurately, minimizing the chances of rejection due to clerical errors. Dr. Kim's practice saw a substantial improvement in the speed of claim processing after adopting such a system. The reduction in errors and the streamlined workflow led to faster payments and a healthier cash flow.

Verification of insurance details upfront is another critical strategy. Ensuring that patient information and coverage details are accurate before providing services can prevent delays down the line. Dr. Martinez's practice incorporated a rigorous verification process during patient check-in. This process included confirming insurance details, coverage limits, and obtaining necessary pre-authorizations. By doing so, Dr. Martinez's team minimized the risk of delays due to verification issues, leading to more timely payments.

Handling pre-authorizations efficiently can also reduce delays. Assigning dedicated staff to manage pre-authorizations ensures that these requirements are met promptly. Dr. Johnson, a dermatologist, found that by having a team member specifically responsible for pre-authorizations, the incidence of delayed payments decreased significantly. This dedicated approach allowed for quicker approval times and ensured that procedures could proceed without unnecessary delays.

Staying on top of claim denials is another essential practice. Establishing a system to monitor and manage denied claims can prevent prolonged delays. Dr. Gupta's neurology clinic faced frequent claim denials initially. By implementing a tracking system and assigning a team to address denials, Dr. Gupta was able to reduce the time taken to resolve these issues. This proactive approach not only minimized delays but also improved the clinic's overall reimbursement rate.

Maintaining open communication with insurers is also vital. Building strong relationships with insurance representatives and regularly communicating to resolve issues can expedite the payment process. Dr. Green's ophthalmology practice benefited from establishing direct contacts within insurance companies. Regular communication and prompt resolution of queries led to faster claim processing and reduced delays.

The impact of insurance delays on cash flow cannot be overstated. These delays can create liquidity issues, making it difficult to cover operational expenses like payroll, supplies, and utilities. For Dr. Evans, who runs a small general practice, delays in insurance payments led to cash flow problems that affected his ability to pay staff on time. By implementing the strategies discussed, Dr. Evans was able to stabilize his cash flow, ensuring that operational expenses were covered without interruption.

Inconsistent cash flow due to delays also complicates financial planning. It becomes challenging to create accurate budgets and forecasts when revenue is unpredictable. Dr. Harrison's dental practice faced this issue, leading to difficulties in planning for future investments and growth. By adopting a more systematic approach to managing insurance delays, Dr. Harrison was able to create more reliable financial plans and make informed decisions about expanding his practice.

Increased borrowing costs are another consequence of insurance delays. Practices might need to rely on credit to cover shortfalls, leading to higher interest expenses. Dr. Reed, an internist, found himself frequently using a line of credit to manage cash flow gaps caused by insurance delays. By streamlining his billing process and improving communication with insurers, Dr. Reed reduced his reliance on credit and lowered his overall borrowing costs.

Let's consider some real-world applications and case studies to see how these strategies work in practice. Dr. Lewis, a gastroenterologist, faced significant delays in insurance payments due to verification and pre-authorization issues. By implementing a rigorous verification process and assigning a dedicated staff member to handle pre-authorizations, Dr. Lewis's practice saw a marked improvement in payment times. This change not only improved cash flow but also enhanced the practice's ability to plan for future investments.

Dr. Parker, a surgeon, struggled with frequent claim denials. He established a denial management team that focused on addressing and appealing denied claims promptly. This team's efforts led to a higher success rate in appeals and a reduction in payment delays. The improved cash flow allowed Dr. Parker to invest in new surgical equipment and expand his practice.

Dr. Adams, an endocrinologist, dealt with delays due to administrative backlogs within insurance companies. By building strong relationships with insurance representatives and scheduling regular follow-ups, Dr. Adams managed to expedite the processing of his claims. The resulting improvement in cash flow enabled her to hire additional staff and reduce patient wait times.

In conclusion, dealing with insurance delays requires a proactive and strategic approach. By understanding the causes of delays, implementing effective management strategies, and maintaining open communication with insurers, you can minimize the impact on your cash flow and ensure the financial stability of your practice. Through real-world examples, we've seen that with the right strategies in place, insurance delays can be effectively managed, turning a significant challenge into an opportunity for improved financial health and operational efficiency. So, take control of your insurance delays, implement these strategies, and watch your practice thrive. It's time to turn these challenges into stepping stones for success and drive your practice toward unparalleled financial stability and growth.

CHAPTER 7:

Mastering Rebates and Incentives from Suppliers

Alright, let's get real about an often overlooked but incredibly powerful financial tool: rebates and incentives from suppliers. These aren't just little bonuses or extras; they're strategic levers that can dramatically improve your practice's cash flow and overall financial health. Understanding and leveraging these rebates and incentives can transform the way you manage your finances, turning what might seem like small gains into significant financial advantages.

First, let's dive into the types of rebates and incentives you might encounter in your medical practice. Rebates can come in various forms, such as volume rebates, which reward you for purchasing large quantities of supplies or equipment. The more you buy, the bigger the rebate. For instance, if you purchase a significant amount of medical supplies from a single supplier, they might offer a rebate of 5% on all purchases above a certain threshold. This not only incentivizes bulk buying but also reduces your overall costs.

Another common type is prompt payment discounts. These are incentives for paying your invoices early. Imagine your supplier offers a 2% discount if you pay within 10 days instead of the usual 30 days. Taking advantage of this can lead to substantial savings over time, especially if you're purchasing large volumes regularly. Loyalty incentives are also prevalent. These are rewards for sticking with the same supplier over a long period, which can come in the form of rebates, discounts, or even exclusive deals on new products.

Then there are bundled purchase discounts, which provide reductions in cost when you buy multiple products or services together. For example, purchasing both medical equipment and the accompanying maintenance services from the same supplier might get you a better overall deal. Seasonal promotions are another form of incentives, where suppliers offer discounts or rebates on certain products during specific times of the year, helping you save on necessary purchases.

Understanding these types is crucial, but what's equally important is how you account for these rebates and incentives. Proper accounting practices ensure that these benefits are reflected accurately in your financial statements, providing a clear picture of your financial health. When you receive a rebate, it should be recorded as a reduction in the cost of goods sold, not as revenue. This keeps your financial statements transparent and prevents inflating your income with what are essentially cost savings.

Let's take an example. Suppose your practice purchases $50,000 worth of medical supplies and receives a $2,500 rebate for reaching a volume threshold. Instead of recording the rebate as revenue, you reduce your cost of goods sold by $2,500. This way, your expense reflects the net amount spent, providing a more accurate picture of your operational costs. Similarly, for prompt payment discounts, the discount should reduce the expense account directly related to the purchase.

Effective management of rebates and incentives also requires strategic planning. Incorporating these financial benefits into your planning process means you're not just reacting to savings but actively seeking and negotiating better deals. This proactive approach can significantly enhance your cash flow management.

Consider Dr. Martin, who runs a network of family clinics. He negotiated a volume rebate with his primary supplier, agreeing to purchase all medical supplies for the year upfront to receive a 10% rebate. By strategically timing his purchases and managing inventory efficiently, Dr. Martin not only reduced his supply costs by 10% but also improved his practice's cash flow. This upfront rebate provided the liquidity needed to invest in new diagnostic equipment, enhancing the quality of care and attracting more patients.

Similarly, Dr. Nguyen, who manages a pediatric clinic, took advantage of prompt payment discounts. By closely monitoring her cash flow and prioritizing early payments, she consistently earned a 2% discount on her substantial monthly supply orders. Over the year, these small discounts accumulated, significantly reducing her overall expenses and freeing up cash for other essential investments, like upgrading the clinic's waiting area and expanding service offerings.

The impact of these rebates and incentives on cash flow can be profound. They provide immediate cost savings, reducing the amount of cash needed for operations. This improved liquidity can then be redirected towards other critical areas, such as expanding services, investing in new technology, or simply ensuring a buffer for unforeseen expenses. By strategically managing these incentives, you can enhance your practice's financial resilience and flexibility.

Let's look at a more detailed case study. Dr. Lewis, an ophthalmologist, runs a busy eye care center. He faced high costs for specialized medical supplies and equipment. After analyzing his expenses, he decided to leverage bundled purchase discounts offered by his supplier. By committing to purchasing both the necessary medical supplies and the accompanying maintenance services in bulk, Dr. Lewis secured a 15% discount on the total package. This strategic move not only lowered his costs but also ensured that his equipment was always in top condition, reducing downtime and improving patient satisfaction.

Dr. Lewis didn't stop there. He also negotiated loyalty incentives with the same supplier. By signing a three-year contract, he received additional annual rebates and exclusive access to new product launches at discounted rates. These incentives significantly improved his cash flow, allowing him to hire more staff and reduce patient wait times, further enhancing the reputation and growth of his practice.

In conclusion, mastering the use of rebates and incentives from suppliers isn't just about saving a few dollars here and there. It's about strategically leveraging these opportunities to enhance your practice's financial health and operational efficiency. By understanding the various types of rebates and incentives, implementing proper accounting practices, and incorporating these benefits into your financial planning, you can unlock significant savings and improve cash flow. Whether it's through volume rebates, prompt payment discounts, or loyalty incentives, these financial tools can provide the liquidity needed to invest in growth and innovation. So, take control, negotiate smartly, and watch your practice thrive. Let's turn those supplier incentives into a powerhouse of financial stability and growth, driving your practice to new heights.

CHAPTER 8:

Mastering Investment Income

Alright, let's talk about taking your medical practice's financial game to the next level. You're already running a successful practice, but what if I told you that there's a way to supplement your operational income without seeing more patients or increasing your services? Enter the world of investment income. This is where your money works for you, generating returns that can significantly boost your financial stability and growth. In this chapter, we're going to delve into different types of investments suitable for medical practices, how to manage them effectively, and the accounting practices that ensure you capture every dollar earned.

First off, let's explore the types of investments that can work wonders for your medical practice. We're not just talking about putting money into a savings account here; we're talking about strategic investments that yield significant returns. Real estate is a prime example. Investing in medical office buildings can provide steady rental income while also appreciating in value over time. Imagine owning the building where your practice operates or leasing space to other healthcare providers. This not only secures your operational space but also generates a reliable income stream.

Stocks and bonds are another potent avenue. By investing in the stock market, you can buy shares in companies, potentially earning dividends and benefiting from stock price appreciation. For a more balanced approach, mutual funds and ETFs (Exchange-

Traded Funds) offer diversified portfolios, spreading the risk and providing steady growth over time. Municipal bonds, which are tax-free, and corporate bonds, which offer higher returns but come with more risk, are excellent ways to generate consistent income while preserving capital.

Private equity and venture capital are more aggressive but highly lucrative options. Investing in healthcare startups can yield substantial returns if these companies succeed. Imagine being an early investor in the next big medical technology or breakthrough treatment. While these investments carry more risk, the potential rewards are enormous.

Alternative investments like hedge funds and Real Estate Investment Trusts (REITs) can also diversify your income streams. Hedge funds use complex strategies to achieve high returns, and though they come with higher risks, they can be incredibly profitable. REITs allow you to invest in real estate markets without owning property directly, providing exposure to the real estate sector and yielding dividends.

Now, let's talk about managing these investments. It's not enough to just throw money into various ventures; you need a strategic plan to monitor and grow your investment income. Diversifying your portfolio is crucial. Spread your investments across different asset classes to minimize risk. Don't put all your eggs in one basket. For example, a mix of real estate, stocks, bonds, and alternative investments can provide a balanced approach that maximizes returns while safeguarding against market volatility.

Regularly monitoring your investments is key. Keep a close eye on how each investment is performing and be prepared to make adjustments as needed. Use financial advisors if necessary to get professional insights. Remember, the financial market is dynamic, and staying informed about market trends, economic indicators, and industry news helps you make timely and strategic decisions.

Reinvesting profits is another powerful strategy. Instead of spending your investment income, consider reinvesting it to compound your returns. This approach can significantly increase your wealth over time. Think of it as planting seeds; the more you reinvest, the more substantial your financial harvest will be in the future.

Managing investment income also involves understanding the risks associated with each investment. Balance high-risk investments with low-risk ones to protect your portfolio. For instance, while investing in a high-growth healthcare startup might offer substantial returns, balancing this with more stable investments like municipal bonds can provide financial stability.

Accurate accounting practices are essential for capturing investment returns. When you buy an investment, record it as an asset on your balance sheet. For example, if you purchase $50,000 worth of stocks, debit your investment account and credit cash. This entry keeps your financial records accurate and transparent. When you receive income from investments, such as dividends or interest, record it as income on your profit and loss statement. For instance, if you receive $5,000 in dividends, debit cash and credit investment income. This practice ensures that your income statements reflect the actual financial benefits of your investments.

Recording gains and losses accurately is also critical. When you sell an investment, any gain or loss impacts your net income and overall financial position. For example, if you sell stocks for

$60,000 that you bought for $50,000, you have a $10,000 gain. Debit cash for $60,000, credit the investment account for $50,000, and credit investment gains for $10,000. If you incur a loss, reverse the gain entry. This accurate accounting provides a clear picture of your financial health and informs better decision-making.

Now, let's bring these concepts to life with some real-world examples of successful investment strategies. Dr. Thompson, who runs a multi-specialty clinic, decided to diversify his income streams through strategic investments. He started by purchasing a medical office building, leasing space to other healthcare providers. This investment generated steady rental income, enhancing his cash flow. Dr. Thompson also invested in mutual funds focused on the healthcare sector. These funds provided consistent returns, further boosting his financial position.

Dr. Thompson didn't stop there. He explored private equity by investing in a promising healthcare startup developing innovative diagnostic tools. While this was a higher-risk investment, it paid off significantly as the startup grew and its valuation soared. The returns from this investment allowed Dr. Thompson to expand his clinic, hire additional staff, and offer new services, driving overall growth.

Another example is Dr. Nguyen, who wanted to generate additional income to fund new equipment for her pediatric practice. She invested in municipal bonds, providing tax-free income, and in a venture capital fund focused on healthcare innovations. The municipal bonds provided a steady, reliable income stream, while the venture capital investment offered substantial returns. This dual approach balanced risk and reward, enhancing Dr. Nguyen's financial stability and enabling her to invest in cutting-edge equipment, improving patient care and attracting more clients.

In conclusion, generating investment income is a powerful strategy for supplementing your medical practice's operational income. By exploring various types of investments, managing them strategically, and implementing accurate accounting practices, you can enhance your financial stability and growth. Whether it's through real estate, stocks, bonds, private equity, or alternative investments, these financial tools can provide the additional income needed to invest in your practice's future. So, take control of your financial destiny, make informed investment decisions, and watch your practice thrive. Let's turn your hard-earned dollars into a thriving financial future, driving your practice to new heights and ensuring long-term success.

CHAPTER 9:

Mastering Grants and Donations for Financial Growth

Alright, let's get real about tapping into an often underutilized goldmine for your medical practice: grants and donations. Imagine having an additional stream of funding that doesn't just trickle in but pours into your practice, allowing you to invest in new technologies, enhance patient care, or even expand your facilities without dipping into your operational budget. Grants and donations can be game-changers, providing the financial boost you need to elevate your practice. This chapter is all about understanding where to find these funds, how to secure them, and how to manage them effectively.

First things first, you need to know where to find these treasure troves. Grants and donations come from various sources, each with its own set of criteria and application processes. Government grants are often the most substantial and can fund a wide range of projects, from research to facility upgrades. Think of federal grants from the National Institutes of Health (NIH) or the Department of Health and Human Services (HHS). These are significant sources, but you have to navigate through their stringent requirements and detailed application processes. State and local grants might be smaller, but they are often easier to obtain and focus on community health initiatives, which can be a perfect fit for many practices.

Private foundations are another goldmine. Organizations like the Robert Wood Johnson Foundation or the Bill & Melinda Gates Foundation provide substantial funding for health-related projects. These foundations are looking to make a significant impact, and if your project aligns with their mission, you could receive significant financial support. Local community foundations also offer grants that support health and wellness initiatives within your community, often with fewer hoops to jump through compared to federal grants.

Corporate donations can also be a substantial source of funding. Many companies have Corporate Social Responsibility (CSR) programs that fund healthcare initiatives. Partnering with these companies can provide both funding and additional resources. Pharmaceutical and medical device companies often fund research and community health programs, promoting their products and services while supporting valuable health projects.

Then, there are individual donors. High-net-worth individuals passionate about healthcare can be a significant source of donations. Crowdfunding platforms like GoFundMe or Kickstarter can also help raise funds for specific projects or equipment. This grassroots approach can engage your community and provide a steady stream of donations for targeted needs.

Once you've identified potential sources of grants and donations, the next step is managing these funds effectively. Securing grants and donations is just the beginning. Effective management ensures that these funds are used optimally and transparently. Start by creating a dedicated fund for grant and donation money. This means setting up a separate account to ensure these funds are not mixed with your operational income.

This segregation makes tracking and reporting easier, providing a clear picture of how these funds are used.

Detailed budgeting is crucial. Develop a comprehensive budget that outlines how the funds will be used. This should include specific line items and projected expenses, ensuring the funds are allocated appropriately. Adhering to the grant's requirements is essential, as most funders require detailed reports on how their money is being used. Maintain meticulous records and be prepared to provide these reports on time.

Regular audits are another critical component of managing grants and donations. Conducting regular internal audits ensures the funds are being used as intended and builds trust with your funders. This transparency is vital for maintaining good relationships with donors and securing future funding.

Accurate accounting is also crucial for managing grants and donations effectively. When you receive a grant or donation, it should be recorded as income. However, if the funds are restricted for specific uses, categorize them accordingly. For example, if you receive a $50,000 grant for purchasing new medical equipment, record it as restricted income. This ensures your financial statements reflect the true nature of the funds and provide transparency.

Tracking expenditures related to the grant or donation separately is also important. This makes it easier to report back to funders and ensures compliance with their requirements. Prepare periodic financial reports that detail how the funds were used and the outcomes achieved. These reports should include a financial summary, outcome metrics, and future projections. This level of detail not only satisfies funder requirements but also demonstrates your practice's commitment to transparency and effective use of funds.

Now, let's bring this to life with some real-world examples of how medical practices have successfully utilized grants and donations. Dr. Rivera runs a community health clinic that serves a low-income population. She identified a need for better prenatal care services but lacked the funds to implement the program. By applying for and receiving a federal grant from the HHS, as well as securing a donation from a local foundation focused on maternal health, Dr. Rivera was able to expand her clinic's services. The grant and donation funded comprehensive prenatal care, including regular check-ups, nutritional counseling, and childbirth classes. This expansion led to a significant reduction in preterm births and improved maternal health in the community.

Another example is Dr. Kim, who runs a research facility focused on innovative cancer treatments. To expand her research capabilities, she needed additional funding for advanced equipment. By partnering with a pharmaceutical company interested in her research area, she secured a substantial donation to fund new equipment. Additionally, she launched a crowdfunding campaign to engage the public and raise additional funds. The new equipment allowed Dr. Kim to conduct cutting-edge research, leading to breakthroughs in cancer treatment. The crowdfunding campaign also raised awareness and support for her research, leading to additional donations and partnerships.

In conclusion, grants and donations are powerful tools that can provide the financial boost your medical practice needs to grow and thrive. By understanding where to find these funds, managing them effectively, and maintaining accurate records, you can leverage these resources to achieve your goals. Whether you're looking to expand services, invest in new equipment, or fund groundbreaking research, grants and donations can make it possible. So, go out there, secure those funds, and take your practice to the next level. Let's turn those opportunities into successes and build a brighter future for your practice and your patients!

CHAPTER 10:

Mastering the Advantages of Leasing Equipment

Let's dive into a strategy that can significantly boost your financial flexibility and operational efficiency: leasing equipment. Imagine having access to the latest medical technology without the hefty upfront costs, and with the ability to upgrade as innovations come along. That's the power of leasing. This approach can positively impact your cash flow, allowing you to allocate resources more effectively and keep your practice at the cutting edge of medical advancements.

Leasing equipment instead of purchasing it outright offers numerous benefits that can transform how your practice operates. First and foremost, leasing helps preserve your cash flow. When you lease, you avoid the significant capital outlay required to purchase expensive medical equipment. Instead, you make manageable monthly payments, which frees up cash for other critical needs, such as staffing, marketing, or expanding your practice. Imagine starting the year with a budget that includes a $300,000 expenditure for new imaging equipment. By leasing instead, that $300,000 stays in your bank account, available for other strategic investments.

Leasing also provides the flexibility to stay current with the latest technology. Medical technology evolves rapidly, and what's state-of-the-art today may be outdated in a few years. Leasing allows you to upgrade your equipment more frequently, ensuring that you always have access to the best tools to provide top-notch patient care. For example, Dr. Patel, who runs a busy cardiology clinic, opted to lease the latest diagnostic equipment. When newer, more advanced models were released two years later, he could easily upgrade without the financial strain of purchasing new equipment outright.

Another advantage of leasing is the potential for maintenance and repair services included in the lease agreement. This can save your practice from unexpected repair costs and downtime. Leasing agreements often come with comprehensive maintenance packages, ensuring that your equipment stays in optimal condition and any issues are promptly addressed. Dr. Lee's pediatric practice benefited from this when her leased ultrasound machine required repairs. The leasing company handled everything, minimizing disruption to her practice and saving her thousands in repair costs.

Now, let's talk about accounting for leased equipment. Proper accounting ensures transparency and accuracy in your financial statements. When you lease equipment, it's recorded differently than when you purchase it. Operating leases, which are more common, do not appear as an asset on your balance sheet. Instead, the lease payments are recorded as an operating expense. This keeps your liabilities lower and can improve financial ratios that potential lenders or investors might consider.

For example, let's say Dr. Martinez leases a new MRI machine for $5,000 per month. Each payment is recorded as a lease expense, which reduces the practice's taxable income. This method provides a clear view of operational expenses without inflating the balance sheet with a large, depreciating asset. If the lease qualifies as a capital lease, it would be treated more like a loan. The equipment would appear as an asset, and the lease obligation as a liability. This type of lease might affect financial ratios differently but can still be advantageous depending on your practice's financial strategy.

The impact of leasing on cash flow is profound. By spreading the cost of equipment over several years, leasing improves cash flow predictability and stability. This predictable expense allows for better financial planning and budgeting. Dr. Nguyen, who manages a dental practice, found that leasing her new digital X-ray machine improved her cash flow significantly. Instead of depleting her reserves, she could manage her monthly expenses more effectively, keeping a buffer for unexpected costs and opportunities for growth.

Real-world examples illustrate the practical benefits of leasing. Dr. Thompson, an orthopedic surgeon, needed to upgrade his surgical equipment to stay competitive. Instead of purchasing, he chose to lease the equipment. This decision allowed him to preserve his capital and invest in marketing initiatives that attracted more patients. The increased patient flow more than covered the lease payments, and his practice grew rapidly.

Another example is Dr. Johnson's dermatology clinic. Facing a tight budget, Dr. Johnson needed new laser treatment equipment but couldn't afford the upfront purchase cost. Leasing provided a solution. By leasing the laser, Dr. Johnson managed to expand her service offerings without financial strain. The predictable monthly lease payments made budgeting easier, and the new services generated additional revenue, improving the clinic's overall profitability.

Dr. Garcia's radiology center also leveraged the benefits of leasing. The center required state-of-the-art imaging equipment to maintain its reputation for high-quality diagnostics. Purchasing the equipment outright would have meant a significant financial outlay, limiting the center's ability to invest in other areas. Instead, Dr. Garcia chose to lease the equipment, which included a full maintenance package. This not only ensured continuous operation with minimal downtime but also kept the center's technology current without the need for massive capital investments every few years.

In conclusion, leasing equipment can be a game-changer for your medical practice. It preserves cash flow, provides flexibility to stay updated with the latest technology, and often includes maintenance and repair services. Proper accounting for leases ensures financial transparency and can improve your financial ratios. By leveraging the advantages of leasing, you can keep your practice financially agile, invest in growth opportunities, and maintain the highest standards of patient care. So, consider leasing as a strategic financial tool and watch your practice thrive with improved cash flow and access to the best medical technology. Let's turn those leasing agreements into catalysts for growth and take your practice to the next level.

CHAPTER 11:

Mastering Deferred Tax Liabilities for Financial Success

Alright, let's dive into a topic that can seem complex but is absolutely crucial for the financial health of your medical practice: deferred tax liabilities. Picture this: you're running a successful practice, but hidden in the shadows of your balance sheet are deferred tax liabilities waiting to impact your future cash flow. Understanding and managing these liabilities effectively can make a significant difference in your financial planning and overall stability. So, let's break down what deferred tax liabilities are, how to account for them, and their impact on your cash flow.

Deferred tax liabilities arise from temporary differences between the income recognized on your financial statements and the income recognized by tax authorities. Think of it as the taxman saying, "I'll collect what's due, but I'll do it later." These liabilities occur when there are differences in timing between when income is earned and when it is taxed. For instance, if your practice uses accelerated depreciation for tax purposes but straight-line depreciation for financial reporting, this creates a temporary difference that results in a deferred tax liability.

To truly grasp the concept, let's consider Dr. Stevens, who operates a thriving dental practice. Dr. Stevens invested in new dental equipment, taking advantage of accelerated depreciation for tax purposes to reduce his taxable income. However, for financial reporting, he uses straight-line depreciation, which spreads the expense evenly over the equipment's useful life. This difference means that while he enjoys lower taxes now, he will face higher taxes later as the temporary difference reverses.

Accounting for deferred tax liabilities requires precision and a keen understanding of tax regulations. When you identify a temporary difference that results in a deferred tax liability, you need to record it on your balance sheet. Let's say Dr. Stevens's accelerated depreciation resulted in a $10,000 tax savings this year. This amount is not a permanent saving but a deferral. To account for this, Dr. Stevens's accountant would record a deferred tax liability of $10,000 on the balance sheet. This entry acknowledges that while the practice benefits from lower taxes now, it will owe more taxes in the future when the temporary difference reverses.

The impact of deferred tax liabilities on cash flow is significant. Initially, these liabilities can provide a boost to your cash flow by reducing your current tax payments. This means more cash on hand to invest in your practice, whether it's upgrading equipment, hiring new staff, or expanding services. However, it's crucial to remember that this benefit is temporary. As the deferred tax liabilities reverse, your future tax payments will increase, impacting your cash flow down the line.

Dr. Stevens understands this dynamic and plans accordingly. By projecting his future tax liabilities, he ensures that he sets aside sufficient funds to cover these future payments. This proactive approach prevents any surprises and maintains the financial stability of his practice. For example, Dr. Stevens creates a financial plan that accounts for the anticipated reversal of his deferred tax liabilities over the next five years. This plan includes setting aside a portion of his current cash flow into a reserve fund dedicated to covering future tax payments. By doing so, he mitigates the risk of a cash flow crunch when the liabilities come due.

Let's delve into some real-world examples to see how effective management of deferred tax liabilities plays out. Dr. Martinez, an orthopedic surgeon, faced a significant deferred tax liability after purchasing state-of-the-art surgical equipment. By using accelerated depreciation, he reduced his current tax burden significantly. However, understanding the implications of deferred taxes, Dr. Martinez worked with his accountant to develop a comprehensive financial plan. This plan included detailed projections of future tax payments and a strategy to set aside funds gradually to cover these payments. As a result, when the deferred tax liabilities began to reverse, Dr. Martinez's practice was well-prepared, avoiding any disruption to his cash flow and maintaining financial stability.

Another example is Dr. Kim, who runs a busy pediatric clinic. She faced deferred tax liabilities due to differences in revenue recognition between her financial statements and tax filings. Dr. Kim's clinic received several large grants, which were recognized as income for tax purposes immediately but deferred for financial reporting. This created a significant deferred tax liability. By working closely with her financial advisor, Dr. Kim developed a strategy to manage these liabilities effectively. She created a reserve fund, setting aside a portion of the grant money to cover future tax payments. This proactive approach ensured that her clinic could continue to operate smoothly without financial strain when the deferred taxes came due.

In conclusion, managing deferred tax liabilities is a critical aspect of financial planning for your medical practice. Understanding these liabilities, implementing accurate accounting practices, and proactively planning for future tax payments can significantly impact your cash flow and financial stability. By recognizing the temporary nature of the benefits provided by deferred tax liabilities and setting aside funds to cover future payments, you can maintain a healthy cash flow and ensure the long-term success of your practice. Just like Dr. Stevens, Dr. Martinez, and Dr. Kim, you can turn deferred tax liabilities from a potential financial burden into a manageable aspect of your financial strategy. Let's take control of these liabilities, plan for the future, and drive your practice toward financial success and stability.

CHAPTER 12:

Mastering Partnership Distributions for Financial Success

Alright, let's talk about a critical aspect of running a successful medical practice with partners: managing partnership distributions. This is one area that can either create harmony and financial stability or lead to confusion and disputes if not handled correctly. Picture this: you and your partners are working hard, growing the practice, and generating income. But how do you ensure that the income is distributed fairly and transparently? How do you account for these distributions, and what impact do they have on your cash flow? Let's dive deep into understanding and mastering partnership distributions to ensure everyone is on the same page and the practice thrives.

First, let's get clear on what partnership distributions are. In a medical practice, income distributed to partners isn't your regular salary. It's the share of the profits after all expenses have been accounted for. It's what you and your partners take home from the practice's earnings. This income is not immediately apparent in cash flow statements because it's derived from the net income of the practice, which only becomes clear after all operational expenses, taxes, and other liabilities are taken care of.

To manage partnership distributions effectively, you must first understand the various types of distributions. Guaranteed payments are one such type, providing a fixed income to partners regardless of the practice's profitability. These are crucial for ensuring that each partner has a baseline income they can rely on, even if the practice has a lean month. For instance, Dr. Stevens, who runs a thriving dental practice with two partners, ensures that each partner receives a guaranteed payment of $10,000 monthly. This amount is recorded as an expense, reducing the practice's net income before profit distributions are calculated.

Profit distributions, on the other hand, are variable and depend entirely on the practice's performance. These distributions are calculated after all expenses and guaranteed payments have been accounted for. If Dr. Stevens's practice generates $150,000 in net income for the quarter after expenses, this amount is split among the partners according to their ownership percentage or as per the partnership agreement. In this case, if the profits are split equally among the three partners, each would receive $50,000.

Accounting for these distributions is where many practices stumble. Proper accounting ensures transparency and fairness, preventing disputes and ensuring everyone understands how the income is divided. For guaranteed payments, these are treated as operating expenses and recorded on the income statement, reducing the net income before profit sharing. For example, Dr. Stevens's accountant would debit the guaranteed payments expense and credit cash each month, reflecting the payout.

When it comes to profit distributions, the process involves recording the distributions on the balance sheet. After calculating the net income, the remaining profit is distributed among partners as per the agreement. Let's say Dr. Stevens's practice has a net income of $300,000 for the year, and it's to be split equally among the three partners. The accountant would debit retained earnings and credit each partner's capital account with $100,000. This process ensures the financial statements accurately reflect the distribution of profits and the reduction in retained earnings.

The impact of partnership distributions on cash flow is significant. While guaranteed payments provide predictable, regular expenses that you can budget for, profit distributions require careful management of cash reserves. Distributing too much can strain your cash flow, especially if the practice faces unexpected expenses or a downturn in revenue. It's essential to balance the desire for immediate profit distribution with the need to maintain sufficient cash reserves for operational stability.

Consider Dr. Thompson's orthopedic clinic, which struggled with uneven cash flow due to unpredictable profit distributions. To address this, Dr. Thompson and his partners decided to retain a portion of the profits within the practice, setting aside a percentage of earnings as a reserve fund before distributing the remaining profits. This approach ensured they had a financial cushion for lean periods or unexpected expenses, stabilizing their cash flow and providing a clearer picture of their financial health.

Transparency and communication are key when managing partnership distributions. Regular meetings to review financial statements and discuss the distribution strategy can prevent misunderstandings and ensure that all partners are on the same page. Dr. Lee's pediatric practice, for example, holds quarterly meetings where partners review the financial performance, discuss any financial concerns, and agree on the distribution of profits. This open communication fosters trust and ensures that each partner feels valued and informed about the practice's financial health.

Let's look at some real-world examples of how effective management of partnership distributions can lead to financial stability and growth. Dr. Kim's multi-specialty clinic faced challenges with managing distributions among her six partners. Initially, the practice distributed profits equally, but this led to dissatisfaction as some partners felt their contributions and efforts were not adequately recognized. To address this, Dr. Kim implemented a performance-based distribution model. Each partner received a base guaranteed payment, and additional profit distributions were based on individual performance metrics such as patient volume, revenue generated, and contributions to the clinic's growth. This approach not only incentivized higher performance but also ensured that distributions reflected each partner's efforts and contributions. As a result, the clinic saw increased productivity, higher revenue, and greater satisfaction among partners.

Another example is Dr. Martinez's cardiology practice. With four partners, they initially faced challenges in managing cash flow due to high profit distributions. They decided to create a strategic reserve fund by retaining 20% of the net income before profit distribution. This fund was used for reinvestments, upgrading equipment, and covering unexpected expenses. The remaining profits were then distributed based on each partner's ownership percentage. This strategy not only stabilized their cash flow but also allowed for continuous improvement and growth of the practice. The partners felt secure knowing that there was a financial buffer, and the practice could make strategic investments without financial strain.

In conclusion, managing partnership distributions is a critical aspect of running a successful medical practice. Understanding the different types of distributions, implementing accurate accounting practices, and balancing cash flow needs are essential for maintaining financial stability and ensuring fairness among partners. Regular communication and transparency in financial matters build trust and foster a collaborative environment where all partners feel valued and informed. By mastering partnership distributions, you can ensure that your practice not only thrives financially but also maintains harmony among partners, driving the practice toward sustained success and growth. Just like Dr. Stevens, Dr. Thompson, Dr. Kim, and Dr. Martinez, you can turn partnership distributions from a potential source of conflict into a strategic advantage. Let's take control of our financial destiny, ensure fair and transparent distributions, and elevate our practice to new heights of success.

CHAPTER 13:

Mastering Expense Reimbursements for Financial Efficiency

Alright, let's dive into a topic that might seem mundane but is absolutely crucial for maintaining the financial health and operational efficiency of your medical practice: managing expense reimbursements. Reimbursements for expenses can often slip through the cracks, creating hidden receivables that obscure your true financial picture. If not handled correctly, they can lead to cash flow issues and financial discrepancies. But don't worry, we're going to turn this often-overlooked task into a streamlined process that supports your practice's growth and stability.

First, let's understand the types of expense reimbursements you might encounter in your practice. These can range from travel and conference expenses to office supplies and professional fees. Travel expenses include costs for flights, hotels, and meals when you or your staff attend medical conferences or training sessions. Office supplies and equipment, on the other hand, cover the day-to-day purchases that keep your practice running smoothly, from paper and pens to medical devices and software subscriptions. Then there are professional fees and memberships, which involve costs for renewing professional licenses, attending workshops, and joining medical associations.

Now, let's talk about the nuts and bolts of accounting for these reimbursements. Proper accounting practices ensure transparency and accuracy, preventing financial misstatements and ensuring compliance with tax regulations. When an expense is incurred by an employee or partner and needs to be reimbursed, it should be recorded as an expense in your accounting system immediately. This practice keeps your financial records up to date and reflects the true operational costs of your practice.

For example, if Dr. Smith attends a medical conference and incurs $2,000 in travel expenses, these costs should be recorded as travel expenses when the expenditure is made. Once Dr. Smith submits the receipts for reimbursement, and the payment is processed, the accounts payable should be credited, and cash should be debited to reflect the reimbursement. This dual-entry method ensures that every transaction is accounted for, providing a clear and accurate picture of your financial health.

Effective management of expense reimbursements starts with a clear, documented policy. This policy should outline what expenses are reimbursable, the process for submitting expenses, and the approval workflow. Dr. Lee's pediatric clinic, for instance, implemented a comprehensive expense reimbursement policy that required employees to submit detailed expense reports with receipts attached. The policy also set deadlines for submission and approval, ensuring timely processing and reimbursement.

Automation can significantly streamline the reimbursement process. By adopting an expense management software, Dr. Lee's clinic reduced the administrative burden on her staff and minimized errors. The software allowed employees to submit expenses electronically, automatically categorize expenses, and generate reports for approval. This automation not only improved efficiency but also provided real-time visibility into expense claims, making it easier to manage cash flow and budget effectively.

The impact of expense reimbursements on cash flow can be significant, especially if not managed properly. Delays in processing reimbursements can create a lag between when the expense is incurred and when it's recognized in your cash flow statements. This lag can obscure your financial picture, leading to discrepancies and potential cash flow issues. For example, if several employees attend a costly training program and submit their expense reports late, the practice might face a sudden outflow of cash that wasn't accounted for in the monthly budget.

Dr. Patel's multi-specialty clinic faced similar challenges. To address this, Dr. Patel implemented a monthly reimbursement schedule, ensuring that all expenses were accounted for and reimbursed within a specific timeframe. This regular schedule allowed for better cash flow management and financial planning. Additionally, Dr. Patel's accountant conducted regular audits of expense reports to ensure accuracy and compliance, identifying any discrepancies early and resolving them promptly.

Let's look at some real-world examples of how effective management of expense reimbursements can benefit your practice. Dr. Thompson's orthopedic clinic struggled with managing travel expenses for conferences and training sessions. Employees would often submit expenses months after the fact, leading to cash flow disruptions and financial discrepancies. Dr. Thompson decided to implement a new expense management system that required employees to submit expenses within 30 days of the expenditure. The system also included automated reminders and a streamlined approval process. As a result, the clinic saw a significant improvement in cash flow stability and reduced administrative workload.

Another example is Dr. Nguyen's dental practice. She faced issues with office supply reimbursements, with employees often purchasing supplies out-of-pocket and submitting expenses sporadically. To streamline the process, Dr. Nguyen established a central purchasing system for office supplies, reducing the need for individual reimbursements. For necessary out-of-pocket expenses, she implemented a pre-approval process and monthly reimbursement cycle. This approach not only improved cash flow management but also provided better control over office supply purchases.

Dr. Martinez's cardiology clinic also leveraged effective expense management to enhance financial efficiency. His clinic frequently incurred professional fees for renewing licenses and attending workshops. Dr. Martinez introduced a dedicated fund for professional development expenses, ensuring that these costs were planned for and reimbursed promptly. This proactive approach prevented unexpected cash flow disruptions and ensured that all professional fees were accounted for in the budget.

In conclusion, managing expense reimbursements effectively is essential for maintaining the financial health of your medical practice. By understanding the types of expense reimbursements, implementing clear accounting practices, and adopting efficient management systems, you can ensure transparency and accuracy in your financial records. Regular audits and scheduled reimbursement cycles can further enhance cash flow stability, providing a clear and accurate financial picture. By following the examples of Dr. Lee, Dr. Patel, Dr. Thompson, Dr. Nguyen, and Dr. Martinez, you can turn the often-overlooked task of expense reimbursements into a streamlined process that supports your practice's growth and stability. Let's take control of our expense management, ensure financial clarity, and drive our practice toward success.

CHAPTER 14:

Mastering the Management of Loan Proceeds

Alright, let's get down to business. Managing loan proceeds is a critical skill for any medical practice that wants to grow, expand, and stay competitive. You see, loans are not just about getting some extra cash; they're about strategic financial leverage. When used wisely, loans can propel your practice to new heights. But if mismanaged, they can lead to financial ruin. So, let's dive deep into understanding how to handle loan proceeds effectively and harness their power to boost your practice's financial health.

First, let's talk about the different types of loans available to medical practices. You've got your traditional bank loans, which are great for long-term investments like purchasing real estate or major equipment. These loans typically offer lower interest rates but require significant collateral and a strong credit history. Then there are SBA loans, backed by the Small Business Administration, which are fantastic for smaller practices looking for favorable terms and lower down payments. Equipment financing is another option, where the equipment itself serves as collateral, making it easier to obtain than traditional loans. Lastly, you have lines of credit, which provide flexible, revolving credit that you can draw upon as needed, ideal for managing short-term cash flow needs.

Understanding the type of loan you're dealing with is crucial because it influences how you'll manage and account for those proceeds. Let's break this down. When those loan proceeds hit your account, it's a game changer. But remember, this isn't income; it's a liability. You've got to pay it back. That's why the first step in managing loan proceeds is proper accounting. You need to record the loan as a liability on your balance sheet. This entry recognizes that while you have the cash now, you also have an obligation to repay it.

Let's say you take out a $100,000 loan. Your initial journal entry would be to debit your cash account and credit a loan payable account. This setup keeps your financial statements accurate and transparent. But the real work begins with managing how you use those proceeds. It's all about strategic allocation. Use loan proceeds for investments that generate returns, like upgrading your medical equipment, expanding your facility, or investing in marketing to attract more patients. Avoid using loan funds for day-to-day operational expenses unless it's a line of credit specifically intended for that purpose.

The impact of loan proceeds on cash flow is significant. On the positive side, they provide immediate liquidity, allowing you to make large purchases or investments without depleting your cash reserves. This can be a lifeline during tough times or a boost when you're ready to expand. However, remember that loans come with repayment obligations, and these payments will affect your future cash flow. It's essential to plan for these repayments in your cash flow forecasts to avoid any surprises.

Let's look at some real-world examples to see how effective loan management can play out. Take Dr. Mitchell's dental practice. Dr. Mitchell wanted to expand his clinic to include a new wing for cosmetic dentistry. He secured a $250,000 SBA loan to cover construction costs and new equipment. By carefully managing these proceeds, he allocated funds precisely where needed: $150,000 went to construction, $80,000 to state-of-the-art equipment, and $20,000 to a marketing campaign announcing the new services. Dr. Mitchell ensured that the loan repayments were factored into his monthly cash flow projections. The expansion was a success, attracting new patients and significantly increasing revenue, which comfortably covered the loan repayments.

Another example is Dr. Kim's pediatric clinic. She faced a cash flow crunch due to delayed insurance payments. To manage this, Dr. Kim secured a $50,000 line of credit. Instead of using it all at once, she drew upon the line of credit as needed, ensuring she only borrowed what was necessary to bridge the gap between insurance reimbursements. This prudent use of credit kept her interest expenses low and provided a financial buffer that maintained the clinic's operations smoothly.

Effective loan management isn't just about getting the money; it's about making that money work for you. It requires disciplined accounting, strategic allocation, and diligent cash flow planning. By understanding the nature of your loan, recording it accurately, and using it wisely, you can transform loan proceeds from a simple liability into a powerful asset that drives growth and stability for your practice.

So, there you have it. Loans can be a powerful tool in your financial arsenal if managed correctly. Don't just take out a loan and hope for the best. Plan, allocate, and manage with precision. Use those proceeds to invest in your practice's future, and watch as strategic financial management propels your practice to new heights. Remember, it's not just about borrowing money; it's about leveraging it to create opportunities and drive success. Let's turn those loan proceeds into a catalyst for growth and make your practice the powerhouse it's meant to be.

CHAPTER 15:

Mastering Contributions to Employee Benefit Plans

Alright, let's dive into a critical aspect of running a successful medical practice: managing contributions to employee benefit plans. Whether you're talking about health insurance, retirement plans, or other employee perks, these benefits are crucial for attracting and retaining top talent. However, the timing and management of these contributions can have a significant impact on your cash flow. Let's explore how to handle these contributions effectively, ensuring your practice remains financially healthy while keeping your team motivated and satisfied.

Employee benefit contributions come in various forms, each with its own set of challenges and timing considerations. Health insurance premiums are typically paid monthly, while retirement contributions can be made on a payroll basis or annually. There are also benefits like tuition reimbursement, bonuses, and other perks that may be paid out at different intervals. Understanding the types of benefit contributions and their timing is essential for effective cash flow management.

Take Dr. Williams, who runs a successful dermatology practice. He offers his employees a comprehensive benefits package that includes health insurance, a 401(k) plan, and annual performance bonuses. To manage these benefits without straining his practice's cash flow, Dr. Williams employs a combination of deferred and prefunded contributions. For health insurance, he makes monthly payments, ensuring that the expense is spread out evenly over the year. This approach avoids large, lump-sum payments that could disrupt cash flow.

When it comes to the 401(k) plan, Dr. Williams contributes on a payroll basis, matching employee contributions each pay period. This method aligns the expense with the timing of payroll, making it easier to manage and predict. By integrating retirement contributions into the regular payroll process, Dr. Williams ensures that these expenses are accounted for consistently, reducing the risk of cash flow surprises.

Annual bonuses, on the other hand, are prefunded throughout the year. Dr. Williams sets aside a portion of his monthly revenue into a separate account designated for bonuses. By the end of the year, he has accumulated the necessary funds to pay out the bonuses without impacting his practice's operational cash flow. This strategy not only ensures that the funds are available when needed but also provides a clear picture of the practice's financial obligations.

Accounting for these benefit contributions requires precise and accurate practices. When making monthly health insurance payments, Dr. Williams records the expense as it occurs, ensuring that his financial statements reflect the true cost of providing this benefit. For the 401(k) contributions, each payroll entry includes a debit to the retirement expense account and a credit to cash, reflecting the outflow of funds. This meticulous accounting ensures that the practice's financial statements are accurate and up to date.

Let's delve into some real-world examples to see how effective management of benefit contributions can enhance financial stability and employee satisfaction. Dr. Kim, who runs a busy pediatric clinic, faced challenges with managing the timing of her employee benefit contributions. Initially, she paid her employees' health insurance premiums quarterly, which led to significant cash flow fluctuations. To address this, Dr. Kim switched to monthly payments, spreading the expense more evenly throughout the year. This change stabilized her cash flow, making it easier to manage other operational expenses.

Dr. Kim also implemented a strategy for managing retirement contributions. Instead of making a lump-sum contribution at the end of the year, she started matching employee contributions each pay period. This approach not only aligned the expense with payroll but also encouraged her employees to contribute more to their retirement plans, knowing that their contributions would be matched promptly. The result was increased employee participation in the 401(k) plan and a more predictable cash flow for the practice.

Another example is Dr. Thompson's orthopedic clinic, which offers a tuition reimbursement program for employees pursuing further education. Initially, Dr. Thompson reimbursed tuition expenses as they occurred, leading to unpredictable cash outflows. To manage this more effectively, he introduced a deferred reimbursement plan. Employees submit their tuition receipts at the beginning of the year, and Dr. Thompson sets aside the total expected reimbursement amount into a separate account. Reimbursements are then made quarterly, providing a balance between supporting employee development and maintaining stable cash flow.

In conclusion, managing contributions to employee benefit plans is essential for maintaining financial stability and ensuring employee satisfaction. By understanding the types of benefit contributions, employing strategies like deferred or prefunded contributions, and implementing accurate accounting practices, you can effectively manage these expenses. Following the examples of Dr. Williams, Dr. Kim, and Dr. Thompson, you can stabilize your cash flow, ensure financial clarity, and create a supportive work environment that attracts and retains top talent. Let's take control of our benefit contributions, enhance our financial planning, and drive our practice toward sustained success.

CHAPTER 16:

Mastering Income from Legal Settlements

Let's talk about a unique and sometimes unexpected source of income that can significantly impact your practice's financial health: legal settlements. Unlike your regular operational income, which you earn through services rendered, income from legal settlements comes from resolving disputes or claims in your favor. This type of income can provide a significant boost to your cash flow, but it requires careful management and accounting to ensure it's leveraged effectively. We're going to delve into understanding legal settlement income, how to account for it, and its impact on your cash flow, illustrated with real-world examples to bring these concepts to life.

First, let's understand what legal settlement income is. Legal settlements arise from disputes that are resolved outside of court or from court rulings where one party agrees to compensate another. For a medical practice, these settlements can come from various sources such as malpractice claims, contract disputes, or even class action suits where your practice might be a beneficiary. For instance, Dr. Harris, who runs a network of clinics, received a significant settlement from a pharmaceutical company due to a class action suit involving a medication that had unreported side effects.

When you receive a legal settlement, it's not like your regular income from patient services. This is a non-operational income, which means it's not derived from the day-to-day activities of your practice but from extraordinary events. This distinction is crucial for proper accounting and financial reporting. Treating settlement income like operational revenue can distort your financial statements and give a misleading picture of your practice's performance.

Accounting for legal settlements requires precision and clarity. When you receive a settlement, you need to record it in a way that clearly separates it from your operational income. This ensures that your financial statements reflect the true nature of your income and provide an accurate basis for decision-making. Let's break this down with an example. Dr. Harris received a $500,000 settlement from the pharmaceutical company. His accountant recorded this amount as "Other Income" on the income statement. This classification distinguishes it from revenue generated by patient services and keeps the financial reporting transparent.

Moreover, the settlement amount might not always be straightforward. Sometimes, a portion of the settlement may be designated for specific purposes such as covering legal fees or reimbursing costs associated with the dispute. These designated amounts should be recorded separately to ensure that they are used appropriately and to maintain accurate financial records. For instance, if $50,000 of Dr. Harris's settlement was allocated for legal fees, this amount would be recorded as an offsetting expense against the settlement income, ensuring that the net impact on income is accurately reflected.

The impact of legal settlements on cash flow can be substantial. Receiving a large settlement can provide an immediate boost to your practice's liquidity, allowing you to make investments, pay down debt, or cover unexpected expenses. However, it's important to manage this windfall carefully. A sudden influx of cash can lead to hasty spending decisions if not managed prudently.

Dr. Harris used a portion of his settlement to invest in new medical equipment for his clinics. This strategic investment enhanced the quality of care provided and attracted more patients, thereby increasing operational income. He also allocated a part of the settlement to create a reserve fund for future legal expenses and unexpected costs, ensuring long-term financial stability.

It's also essential to consider the tax implications of legal settlements. Depending on the nature of the settlement, the income may be taxable, and failing to account for this can lead to unexpected tax liabilities. Dr. Harris consulted with his accountant to understand the tax treatment of his settlement. They determined that a portion of the settlement related to lost income was taxable, while another part, intended to cover legal expenses, was not. By accurately accounting for these differences, Dr. Harris was able to plan for his tax obligations and avoid any surprises.

Real-world examples can illustrate the practical aspects of managing legal settlement income effectively. Dr. Lee, a prominent surgeon, received a settlement from a malpractice insurance claim. This settlement was a result of a lengthy legal battle, and the funds were intended to compensate for lost income during the period she was unable to practice. Dr. Lee worked with her financial advisor to ensure the settlement was recorded correctly, distinguishing it from her operational income. This clear accounting allowed her to reinvest a portion of the funds into her practice, upgrading surgical equipment and expanding her clinic's services. The remainder was used to build a financial cushion, providing her with the stability needed to navigate future uncertainties.

Another example is Dr. Martinez, who managed to secure a settlement from a real estate dispute involving the purchase of a new clinic location. The settlement covered not only the legal fees but also compensated for the delays and lost income due to the dispute. Dr. Martinez's careful planning and strategic use of the settlement funds enabled him to complete the purchase and renovation of the new clinic. By recording the settlement as non-operational income and accounting for the associated legal expenses separately, Dr. Martinez maintained a clear financial picture that guided his subsequent business decisions.

In conclusion, managing income from legal settlements requires a nuanced approach that distinguishes it from regular operational income. Proper accounting practices ensure transparency and accuracy, preventing financial misstatements and enabling informed decision-making. The impact on cash flow can be substantial, providing opportunities for investment, debt reduction, and financial stability. By following the examples of Dr. Harris, Dr. Lee, and Dr. Martinez, you can turn legal settlements into a strategic advantage for your practice. Careful management and strategic planning are key to leveraging these funds effectively, ensuring they contribute to your practice's long-term success and stability. Let's take control of our financial destiny, master the management of legal settlement income, and drive our practice toward new heights of success.

CHAPTER 17:

Mastering Non-Operating Income Sources for Financial Growth

Alright, let's dive into a critical yet often overlooked aspect of running a successful medical practice: non-operating income. While your primary revenue comes from patient services, there are numerous opportunities to boost your cash flow through non-operating activities. These are the hidden gems in your financial strategy that can make a significant difference when managed correctly. Think of it as finding money in places you hadn't thought to look before. We're going to explore the various types of non-operating income, how to account for them, and their impact on your cash flow, enriched with real-world examples to illustrate these concepts.

First, let's get clear on what non-operating income is. Non-operating income comes from activities that are not part of your core medical services. This can include selling old equipment, renting out unused property, investment income, or even winning a legal settlement. For instance, Dr. Johnson, who runs a multi-specialty clinic, discovered a substantial non-operating income stream by selling outdated medical equipment when upgrading to newer models. This sale provided a significant cash influx that wasn't part of the regular operational income.

Understanding the types of non-operating income is crucial. Selling old equipment is one of the most straightforward sources. When you upgrade your medical equipment, the old machines don't just have to gather dust or get thrown away. They can be sold to other practices or equipment resellers, generating a tidy sum. For example, Dr. Johnson sold his old MRI machine for $50,000, which he then reinvested into his practice. Another source is selling property. If your practice owns real estate that's no longer in use, selling or leasing it can provide a significant cash boost. Dr. Lee, a pediatrician, sold a small office building that was previously used as a satellite location but had become redundant after consolidating services into a larger facility.

Investment income is another powerful non-operating income source. This includes dividends from stocks, interest from bonds, or returns from other financial investments. Dr. Martinez, an ophthalmologist, had a well-diversified investment portfolio that provided a steady stream of income from dividends and interest. This investment income allowed him to cover unexpected expenses without tapping into the practice's operational funds. Additionally, rental income can be a significant non-operating revenue stream if your practice owns property that can be leased out. Dr. Patel, who runs a dermatology clinic, rented out part of his building to a complementary healthcare provider, creating a steady monthly income.

Accounting for non-operating income is essential to maintain financial transparency and accuracy. When you receive non-operating income, it should be recorded separately from your operational revenue. This ensures that your financial statements reflect the true nature of your income sources and provide an accurate basis for decision-making. For instance, when Dr. Johnson sold his MRI machine, the $50,000 was recorded as "Other Income" on the income statement. This classification distinguished it from revenue generated by patient services, maintaining the clarity of financial reporting.

The impact of non-operating income on cash flow can be substantial. Unlike regular income, which is predictable and recurrent, non-operating income can be irregular and substantial. This influx of cash can provide immediate liquidity, allowing you to invest in new opportunities, pay down debt, or cover unexpected expenses. However, it's important to manage this windfall carefully. A sudden influx of cash can lead to hasty spending decisions if not managed prudently.

Dr. Johnson, after selling his MRI machine, used part of the proceeds to purchase new equipment and allocated a portion to a reserve fund for future upgrades and emergencies. This strategic approach ensured that the non-operating income was used effectively to support the long-term stability and growth of his practice.

Let's delve into some real-world examples to see how effective management of non-operating income can enhance financial stability and growth. Dr. Lee's pediatric practice faced cash flow challenges due to a recent expansion. By selling an old office building that was no longer in use, she generated $300,000 in non-operating income. This sale not only alleviated the immediate cash flow issues but also provided the funds needed to complete the expansion and invest in new medical equipment. Dr. Lee's strategic use of non-operating income transformed a potential financial burden into an opportunity for growth and improvement.

Another example is Dr. Martinez's ophthalmology practice. With a well-diversified investment portfolio, Dr. Martinez received regular dividends and interest income. This non-operating income provided a financial cushion that allowed him to handle unexpected expenses without disrupting the practice's operations. When a major piece of equipment needed urgent replacement, Dr. Martinez used the investment income to cover the cost, ensuring that his practice continued to operate smoothly without financial strain.

Dr. Patel's dermatology clinic also illustrates the benefits of non-operating income. By renting out part of his building to a complementary healthcare provider, Dr. Patel created a steady stream of rental income. This additional revenue not only enhanced his cash flow but also fostered a collaborative environment that benefited both practices. The rental income was recorded separately from the operational revenue, ensuring clear and accurate financial reporting.

In conclusion, non-operating income is a powerful tool for enhancing the financial health and stability of your medical practice. By understanding the types of non-operating income, implementing accurate accounting practices, and strategically managing these funds, you can leverage these opportunities to support your practice's growth and stability. Whether it's selling old equipment, renting out unused property, or generating investment income, these non-operating activities can provide significant financial benefits. Following the examples of Dr. Johnson, Dr. Lee, Dr. Martinez, and Dr. Patel, you can turn non-operating income into a strategic advantage for your practice. Let's take control of our financial destiny, master the management of non-operating income, and drive our practice toward new heights of success.

CHAPTER 18:

Mastering Barter Transactions for Financial Success

Alright, let's talk about a powerful yet often overlooked strategy for enhancing your practice's financial health: barter transactions. Imagine trading your medical services for essential goods or services without a single dollar changing hands. It's like a financial jiu-jitsu move that can boost your cash flow and provide valuable resources without impacting your cash reserves. Barter transactions can be a game-changer if you know how to use them effectively. We're going to break down what barter transactions are, how to account for them, their impact on cash flow, and explore real-world examples that demonstrate their benefits.

First, let's understand what barter transactions are. Barter transactions involve the exchange of goods or services between parties without the use of cash. Instead of paying with money, you offer something of value that the other party needs. For instance, Dr. Thompson, who runs a successful dental practice, might exchange dental services with a marketing firm in return for their expertise in creating a marketing campaign for his practice. No money changes hands, but both parties receive valuable services that help their businesses grow.

Barter transactions can be incredibly beneficial, especially for medical practices. They allow you to access services or goods without dipping into your cash reserves, making it easier to manage your cash flow. Moreover, barter transactions can foster stronger relationships with other local businesses, creating a network of mutual support and collaboration. For Dr. Thompson, trading dental services for marketing expertise not only saved cash but also resulted in a highly effective marketing campaign that attracted new patients.

Now, let's delve into the accounting side of barter transactions. Proper accounting practices are crucial to ensure transparency and accuracy in your financial statements. When engaging in a barter transaction, you need to recognize the fair market value of the goods or services exchanged. This means assigning a monetary value to the services you provide and the services you receive, even though no cash is involved.

For example, if Dr. Thompson agrees to provide $5,000 worth of dental services in exchange for $5,000 worth of marketing services, both the dental services provided and the marketing services received should be recorded at their fair market value. In Dr. Thompson's accounting records, this would be reflected by debiting the marketing expense account and crediting the dental service revenue account. This approach ensures that the transaction is accurately recorded and reflected in the financial statements, providing a clear picture of the practice's economic activities.

Barter transactions can have a significant impact on cash flow. By trading services instead of paying cash, you can preserve your cash reserves for other critical needs. This can be especially beneficial during periods of tight cash flow or when unexpected expenses arise. For instance, if Dr. Thompson's dental practice faces a sudden increase in supply costs, having engaged in barter transactions can ensure that there are sufficient cash reserves to cover these expenses without compromising the practice's financial stability.

Moreover, barter transactions can help you access services that might otherwise be unaffordable. For example, Dr. Lee, who runs a pediatric clinic, needed new furniture for her waiting room but didn't have the budget for it. By bartering medical services with a local furniture store, she was able to furnish her clinic without spending cash. This not only improved the clinic's environment but also attracted more patients, enhancing the practice's reputation and revenue.

Let's explore some real-world examples to see how barter transactions can be effectively utilized. Dr. Martinez, an ophthalmologist, successfully used barter transactions to upgrade his practice's technology. He needed new computer systems but didn't want to deplete his cash reserves. By partnering with a local tech company, Dr. Martinez provided eye care services for the company's employees in exchange for the new computer systems. This transaction allowed him to enhance his practice's technology without impacting his cash flow, while the tech company benefited from comprehensive eye care for its staff.

Another example is Dr. Patel's dermatology clinic, which faced a similar situation. Dr. Patel needed to redesign her clinic's website but had a limited budget. By bartering dermatology services with a web design firm, she was able to get a professional, modern website without spending any cash. The new website attracted more patients and boosted the clinic's online presence, leading to increased revenue. The web design firm, in turn, benefited from Dr. Patel's expert dermatological services.

Dr. Nguyen, a chiropractor, also leveraged barter transactions to grow his practice. He wanted to offer wellness workshops to his patients but didn't have the expertise in-house. By bartering chiropractic services with a local nutritionist and yoga instructor, Dr. Nguyen was able to offer comprehensive wellness workshops that enhanced his patients' experience and loyalty. These workshops attracted new patients and created additional revenue streams, all without impacting his cash reserves.

In conclusion, barter transactions are a powerful tool for enhancing your medical practice's financial health. By understanding how to engage in these transactions, implementing proper accounting practices, and recognizing their impact on cash flow, you can leverage barter to access valuable goods and services without spending cash. Whether it's trading dental services for marketing expertise, medical services for new office furniture, or chiropractic care for wellness workshops, barter transactions can provide significant financial benefits. Following the examples of Dr. Thompson, Dr. Lee, Dr. Martinez, Dr. Patel, and Dr. Nguyen, you can turn barter transactions into a strategic advantage for your practice. Let's take control of our financial destiny, master the art of barter, and drive our practice toward new heights of success.

CHAPTER 19:

Mastering Income from Research Activities

Alright, let's dive into a highly lucrative but often underexplored avenue for boosting your practice's cash flow: income from research activities. Participating in clinical trials or engaging in other research projects can provide a significant additional revenue stream. These activities not only enhance your practice's financial health but also contribute to medical advancements and increase your practice's reputation in the medical community. We're going to break down the types of research activities that generate income, how to manage this income effectively, the best accounting practices, and real-world examples that illustrate successful research income management.

First, let's understand the types of research activities that can generate income. Clinical trials are one of the most common and profitable research activities. Pharmaceutical companies and research institutions frequently seek medical practices to conduct trials for new medications or treatments. For instance, Dr. Thompson, who runs a multi-specialty clinic, partnered with a pharmaceutical company to conduct a clinical trial for a new hypertension drug. This partnership provided his practice with substantial funding in exchange for recruiting patients and administering the trial.

Another lucrative area is collaborative research with academic institutions. Universities and research centers often require the expertise and patient access that medical practices provide. Dr. Lee, a pediatrician, collaborated with a nearby university to study the effects of a new vaccine. This collaboration not only brought in additional income but also enhanced her practice's academic profile and provided cutting-edge treatment options for her patients.

Medical device testing is another source of research income. Companies developing new medical devices need real-world testing environments, making medical practices ideal partners. Dr. Martinez, an ophthalmologist, partnered with a medical device company to test a new type of intraocular lens. This partnership provided significant funding and allowed Dr. Martinez to offer his patients access to the latest technology before it became widely available.

Managing research income requires strategic planning and meticulous organization. When engaging in research activities, it's crucial to have clear contracts that outline the scope of work, payment terms, and responsibilities. For example, Dr. Thompson ensured that his contract with the pharmaceutical company specified the milestones for patient recruitment and the corresponding payments. This clarity helped manage expectations and ensured timely payments.

It's also essential to have a dedicated team or staff member overseeing the research activities. Dr. Lee assigned one of her senior nurses to coordinate the vaccine study, ensuring that all procedures were followed correctly, and data was accurately recorded. This coordination ensured the research ran smoothly and complied with all regulatory requirements.

Now, let's talk about accounting for research income. Accurate accounting practices are crucial to ensure transparency and compliance with financial regulations. When you receive research income, it should be recorded separately from your regular operational income. This distinction helps in providing a clear financial picture and ensures that the income is used appropriately.

For instance, when Dr. Thompson received payments from the pharmaceutical company, his accountant recorded this income under a separate line item called "Research Income." This categorization ensured that the income from the clinical trial was easily identifiable and separate from patient service revenue. Additionally, any expenses related to the research, such as additional staffing or equipment, were recorded as "Research Expenses." This clear accounting practice provided an accurate financial picture and facilitated better financial planning.

It's also important to regularly reconcile the research income and expenses to ensure that all payments are received and accounted for. Dr. Lee's practice conducted monthly reconciliations to match the payments received from the university with the milestones achieved in the vaccine study. This regular review ensured that there were no discrepancies and that the practice was reimbursed for all its efforts.

The impact of research income on cash flow can be significant. Unlike regular patient service revenue, which can be relatively steady, research income can come in larger, less frequent payments. These payments can provide a substantial boost to your cash flow, allowing you to invest in new equipment, hire additional staff, or expand your practice. However, it's essential to manage this income carefully to avoid disruptions.

Dr. Martinez, for example, used the income from the medical device testing to upgrade his clinic's diagnostic equipment. This strategic investment not only improved the quality of care but also attracted more patients, increasing his regular revenue. He also set aside a portion of the research income to create a reserve fund for future research projects or unexpected expenses.

Let's explore some real-world examples of successful research income management. Dr. Patel, who runs a dermatology clinic, participated in several clinical trials for new skincare treatments. By strategically selecting trials that aligned with her clinic's expertise, Dr. Patel was able to generate significant research income. She used this income to renovate her clinic and purchase state-of-the-art equipment, enhancing patient care and attracting high-profile clients. Dr. Patel also reinvested a portion of the research income into further research, creating a cycle of continuous improvement and innovation.

Another example is Dr. Nguyen, a cardiologist who collaborated with a medical school to study the effects of a new heart medication. The research income allowed Dr. Nguyen to expand his clinic and hire additional staff, increasing the clinic's capacity to treat more patients. By maintaining clear accounting practices and regularly reviewing the financials, Dr. Nguyen ensured that the research income was used effectively and contributed to the clinic's growth and stability.

Dr. Johnson's orthopedic clinic also benefited from engaging in research activities. He partnered with a biotech company to test a new joint replacement device. The income from this partnership allowed Dr. Johnson to invest in advanced surgical equipment and training for his staff. The success of the research project not only provided financial benefits but also positioned his clinic as a leader in innovative treatments, attracting more patients and high-value research opportunities.

In conclusion, income from research activities can provide a substantial boost to your medical practice's cash flow. By understanding the types of research activities that generate income, managing the income effectively, and implementing accurate accounting practices, you can leverage these opportunities to support your practice's growth and stability. Whether it's participating in clinical trials, collaborating with academic institutions, or testing new medical devices, research activities offer significant financial and professional benefits. Following the examples of Dr. Thompson, Dr. Lee, Dr. Martinez, Dr. Patel, Dr. Nguyen, and Dr. Johnson, you can turn research income into a strategic advantage for your practice. Let's take control of our financial destiny, master the management of research income, and drive our practice toward new heights of success.

CHAPTER 20:

Mastering Vendor Financing Arrangements for Financial Flexibility

Alright, let's get into a savvy financial strategy that can significantly improve your practice's cash flow and overall financial health: vendor financing arrangements. Picture this: you need new medical equipment, but instead of paying upfront, the vendor allows you to finance the purchase. This means you get the necessary tools to enhance patient care and grow your practice without an immediate cash outflow. Vendor financing can be a game-changer if managed correctly. We're going to delve into understanding vendor financing, how to manage these agreements effectively, the best accounting practices, and practical examples that illustrate the benefits of vendor financing.

First, let's break down what vendor financing is. Vendor financing is a financing arrangement where the vendor—usually a supplier of equipment or services—provides financing to the buyer. Instead of paying the full amount upfront, the buyer agrees to make payments over time. This can include payment plans, deferred payments, or even loans provided directly by the vendor. For a medical practice, this means acquiring essential equipment without depleting your cash reserves.

Dr. Thompson, who runs a multi-specialty clinic, needed to upgrade his diagnostic equipment but didn't have the available cash flow for such a significant expenditure. By entering into a vendor financing arrangement with the equipment supplier, he was able to get the necessary tools immediately and pay for them over a three-year period. This not only allowed him to enhance patient care but also kept his cash flow stable.

Managing vendor financing agreements requires careful planning and negotiation. It's essential to thoroughly understand the terms of the agreement, including the interest rate, payment schedule, and any penalties for late payments. For example, when Dr. Thompson negotiated his vendor financing agreement, he ensured that the interest rate was competitive and that the payment schedule aligned with his practice's cash flow patterns. He also negotiated a grace period for the first payment, giving his practice time to generate additional revenue from the new equipment before the payments began.

Clear communication with the vendor is crucial throughout the financing period. Regularly reviewing the terms and ensuring timely payments can prevent misunderstandings and maintain a positive relationship with the supplier. Dr. Lee, a pediatrician, set up automated payments for her vendor financing agreement, ensuring that payments were made on time and reducing the administrative burden on her staff. This approach not only maintained a good relationship with the vendor but also avoided any late payment penalties.

Now, let's talk about the accounting practices for vendor financing. Accurate accounting is essential to ensure transparency and maintain a clear financial picture. When you enter into a vendor financing agreement, it's important to record the liability accurately on your balance sheet. This means recognizing the full amount of the purchase as a liability, even though the payments will be made over time.

For instance, Dr. Thompson's accountant recorded the full cost of the new diagnostic equipment as a liability when the vendor financing agreement was signed. Each payment made reduced the liability and was recorded as an expense on the income statement. This approach ensured that the practice's financial statements accurately reflected the outstanding obligation and the ongoing cost of the equipment.

The impact of vendor financing on cash flow can be significant. By spreading the cost of a major purchase over several years, you can preserve your cash reserves for other critical needs, such as staffing, marketing, or unexpected expenses. Dr. Martinez, an ophthalmologist, used vendor financing to acquire a state-of-the-art laser system. The financing arrangement allowed him to keep his cash reserves intact while benefiting from the immediate use of the new technology. This improved his practice's competitive edge and attracted more patients, ultimately increasing his revenue.

Vendor financing can also provide financial flexibility during periods of growth or expansion. Dr. Patel's dermatology clinic experienced rapid growth, necessitating the purchase of additional equipment and expansion of facilities. By leveraging vendor financing, Dr. Patel was able to manage the cash outflow effectively, ensuring that the practice could continue to grow without financial strain. The predictable monthly payments made budgeting easier and allowed for strategic planning.

Let's explore some real-world examples of successful vendor financing arrangements. Dr. Nguyen, who runs a busy dental practice, needed to upgrade her practice management software to streamline operations and improve patient care. The upfront cost was substantial, but the software vendor offered a financing arrangement that spread the payments over five years. This allowed Dr. Nguyen to implement the new system immediately, enhancing efficiency and patient satisfaction without impacting her cash flow. The improved operational efficiency led to cost savings and increased revenue, making the financing arrangement a strategic investment.

Another example is Dr. Johnson's orthopedic clinic, which required new surgical equipment to keep up with advancements in medical technology. By negotiating a vendor financing agreement with the equipment supplier, Dr. Johnson was able to acquire the latest surgical tools without a significant upfront expenditure. The financing terms included a low-interest rate and flexible payment schedule, aligning with the clinic's cash flow patterns. This arrangement not only provided immediate access to cutting-edge technology but also supported the clinic's financial stability and growth.

In conclusion, vendor financing arrangements can be a powerful tool for enhancing your medical practice's financial flexibility and growth. By understanding the terms of the agreement, managing the financing effectively, and implementing accurate accounting practices, you can leverage vendor financing to acquire essential equipment and services without impacting your cash flow. Whether it's upgrading diagnostic equipment, expanding facilities, or implementing new software, vendor financing can provide significant financial benefits. Following the examples of Dr. Thompson, Dr. Lee, Dr. Martinez, Dr. Patel, Dr.

Nguyen, and Dr. Johnson, you can turn vendor financing into a strategic advantage for your practice. Let's take control of our financial destiny, master the management of vendor financing arrangements, and drive our practice toward new heights of success.

CHAPTER 21:

Mastering Delayed Recognition of Credit Card Payments

Alright, let's dive into a topic that can be a real headache for any medical practice: delayed recognition of credit card payments. Imagine this: you provide top-notch care, your patients swipe their cards, but the money doesn't hit your account right away. The lag in processing times can mess with your cash flow, making it harder to manage your finances and keep everything running smoothly. But don't worry, I'm going to show you how to navigate these delays like a pro, ensuring that your practice stays financially healthy and stable.

First, let's understand the challenges posed by delayed credit card payments. When a patient pays with a credit card, the transaction has to go through several steps before the money lands in your bank account. It's not instantaneous. The payment has to be authorized, then processed by the credit card network, and finally settled by your merchant bank. Each step can introduce delays, and sometimes, it can take several days before you see the funds. This delay can disrupt your cash flow, especially if a significant portion of your revenue comes from credit card payments.

Dr. Stevens, who runs a bustling dermatology clinic, often found himself in a bind because of these delays. His patients preferred paying with credit cards, but the lag in receiving the funds meant that he sometimes struggled to cover immediate expenses like payroll, supplies, and rent. This scenario is common in many practices, and managing these delays is crucial to maintaining financial stability.

To effectively manage payment delays, it's essential to have a clear understanding of your payment processing timeline. Knowing how long it typically takes for credit card payments to be processed and settled can help you plan better. Dr. Stevens began by closely monitoring his payment processor's timeline. He found that, on average, it took three days for payments to be deposited into his account. With this information, he could better forecast his cash flow and plan for periods when funds might be tight.

One effective strategy is to maintain a cash reserve that can cover your operating expenses during these delays. Dr. Stevens set up a reserve fund specifically for this purpose. By keeping an amount equivalent to at least a week's worth of operating expenses in reserve, he ensured that his clinic could continue to function smoothly even if there was a delay in receiving credit card payments. This buffer allowed him to manage his cash flow more effectively and avoid any financial hiccups.

Regular reconciliation of your credit card transactions is also critical. By matching the transactions recorded in your accounting system with the deposits made to your bank account, you can quickly identify any discrepancies or issues. Dr. Stevens's accountant performed daily reconciliations to ensure that all credit card payments were accounted for accurately. This practice helped them catch any missing or delayed payments early, allowing them to address issues promptly with the payment processor.

Accurate accounting practices are essential for managing delayed credit card payments. When a credit card payment is made, it should be recorded as accounts receivable until the funds are actually deposited into your account. Once the payment is settled and the money is in your bank account, you can then convert it from accounts receivable to cash. This method ensures that your financial statements accurately reflect the timing of your income and expenses.

For instance, when Dr. Stevens's clinic receives a credit card payment, his accountant records the transaction as an increase in accounts receivable. Once the payment is settled and deposited, the accountant then records it as cash in the bank, reducing the accounts receivable balance. This approach provides a clear and accurate picture of the clinic's financial position, even if there are delays in receiving the funds.

Let's explore some real-world examples of how effective management of delayed credit card payments can benefit your practice. Dr. Kim, a pediatrician, faced similar challenges with delayed payments. By negotiating better terms with her payment processor, she was able to reduce the average processing time from four days to two days. This improvement had a significant positive impact on her cash flow, allowing her to invest in new equipment and expand her clinic's services.

Another example is Dr. Patel's dental practice, which implemented a more robust accounting system to manage delayed payments. By integrating their practice management software with their accounting system, they could automatically track credit card transactions and reconcile them daily. This automation reduced the administrative burden on the staff and ensured that all payments were accounted for accurately and promptly. As a result, Dr. Patel's practice saw improved cash flow management and greater financial stability.

In conclusion, managing delayed recognition of credit card payments is crucial for maintaining the financial health of your medical practice. By understanding the challenges posed by payment delays, implementing strategies to manage these delays, and adopting accurate accounting practices, you can navigate these issues effectively. Following the examples of Dr. Stevens, Dr. Kim, and Dr. Patel, you can turn the challenge of delayed credit card payments into a manageable aspect of your financial strategy. Let's take control of our cash flow, master the management of delayed payments, and drive our practice toward new heights of financial success.

CHAPTER 22:

Mastering Deferred Revenue from Subscription Services

Alright, let's talk about a powerful financial strategy that can significantly stabilize and boost your practice's revenue: subscription-based services. Imagine setting up a steady stream of income that flows in regularly, providing financial stability and predictability. However, there's a twist—while you bill your patients periodically, the revenue is recognized over time. This creates deferred revenue, which, if managed correctly, can be a game-changer for your cash flow and overall financial health. We're going to explore what deferred revenue is, how to manage subscription services effectively, the accounting practices you need to adopt, and real-world examples to bring these concepts to life.

First, let's understand what deferred revenue is. Deferred revenue, also known as unearned revenue, is money received by a business for goods or services yet to be delivered. In the context of a medical practice, this often applies to subscription-based services, where patients pay upfront for services to be provided over a period of time. For instance, Dr. Stevens, who runs a successful dermatology clinic, offers a skincare subscription service. Patients pay an annual fee for quarterly treatments and continuous skincare products. Even though the clinic receives the payment upfront, the revenue is only recognized as each treatment is delivered.

Managing subscription services requires a strategic approach. It's not just about getting patients to sign up; it's about ensuring they see the value in their subscription and remain committed over time. Dr. Stevens's clinic achieves this by offering personalized skincare plans, regular check-ins, and exclusive access to new products. This level of service keeps patients engaged and reduces the likelihood of cancellations, ensuring a steady stream of income.

Effective communication is key to managing subscriptions. Patients need to understand what they're getting, how often they'll receive services, and the benefits of staying subscribed. Dr. Stevens's team sends regular updates, reminding patients of upcoming appointments and new product releases, maintaining a high level of engagement and satisfaction. This proactive approach not only enhances patient experience but also ensures that the clinic consistently delivers on its promises, thereby avoiding any disruptions in revenue recognition.

Now, let's dive into the accounting practices for managing deferred revenue. Accurate accounting is crucial to reflect the true financial health of your practice. When you receive payment for a subscription service, it should initially be recorded as deferred revenue, a liability on your balance sheet. This approach acknowledges that while you have the cash, you haven't yet earned it because the service hasn't been fully delivered.

For example, if Dr. Stevens's clinic receives $1,200 from a patient for an annual skincare subscription, the full amount is recorded as deferred revenue at the time of payment. As each quarterly treatment is provided, a portion of this deferred revenue is recognized as earned revenue. So, after the first treatment, $300 is transferred from deferred revenue to earned revenue. This process continues until the entire subscription fee is recognized as earned revenue over the year.

The impact of deferred revenue on cash flow can be substantial. Receiving the full payment upfront boosts your cash reserves, allowing you to invest in your practice, cover operating expenses, or handle unexpected costs. However, it's essential to manage this cash responsibly, knowing that the revenue is recognized over time. Dr. Stevens uses a portion of the upfront payments to invest in new equipment and training for his staff, ensuring that the clinic continues to deliver high-quality services. The rest is allocated to a reserve fund to cover any operational costs that arise before the revenue is fully recognized.

Let's explore some real-world examples to see how effective management of deferred revenue can benefit your practice. Dr. Kim, a pediatrician, introduced a wellness subscription service for her young patients. Parents pay an annual fee that covers regular check-ups, vaccinations, and telehealth consultations. By offering a comprehensive package, Dr. Kim ensures consistent cash flow while providing valuable services that keep her patients healthy and their parents satisfied.

Dr. Kim's accountant records the full subscription fee as deferred revenue and gradually recognizes it as services are rendered. This accurate accounting ensures that the practice's financial statements reflect the true state of its finances. With the upfront payments, Dr. Kim invested in new telehealth technology, enhancing her service offerings and attracting more subscribers.

This strategic investment not only improved patient care but also boosted the practice's reputation and revenue.

Another example is Dr. Patel's dental practice, which offers a dental care subscription. Patients pay monthly fees for regular cleanings, exams, and discounts on other services. This model provides a steady stream of income and encourages patients to maintain regular dental care, reducing the likelihood of major dental issues. Dr. Patel's practice records the monthly payments as deferred revenue and recognizes it as each service is provided. This approach ensures a consistent flow of recognized revenue, supporting the practice's cash flow and financial stability.

Dr. Martinez, an ophthalmologist, leveraged subscription services to offer a vision care package that includes annual exams, prescription updates, and discounts on eyewear. Patients appreciate the convenience and savings, leading to high subscription renewal rates. The upfront payments are recorded as deferred revenue, and as services are delivered, the revenue is recognized. This method not only stabilizes cash flow but also allows Dr. Martinez to plan for future investments in advanced diagnostic equipment and expanded services.

In conclusion, managing deferred revenue from subscription services is a powerful strategy for enhancing the financial health and stability of your medical practice. By understanding the nature of deferred revenue, implementing effective management strategies, and adopting accurate accounting practices, you can leverage subscription services to create a steady and predictable income stream. Whether it's offering skincare packages, wellness subscriptions, dental care plans, or vision care packages, subscription services provide significant financial benefits.

Following the examples of Dr. Stevens, Dr. Kim, Dr. Patel, and Dr. Martinez, you can turn deferred revenue into a strategic advantage for your practice. Let's take control of our financial destiny, master the management of subscription services, and drive our practice toward new heights of success.

CHAPTER 23:

Mastering Advance Payments for Future Services

Alright, let's get into a financial strategy that can give your practice a significant boost in stability and predictability: advance payments for future services. Imagine this: your patients trust you so much that they're willing to pay for your services upfront, providing you with an immediate influx of cash. This scenario is a dream for many practices because it ensures a steady stream of revenue and reduces the stress of daily cash flow management. However, it's crucial to handle these advance payments correctly, as they initially represent liabilities on your balance sheet. We're going to explore the different types of advance payments, how to manage them effectively, the necessary accounting practices, and real-world examples to illustrate these concepts.

First, let's understand what advance payments are. These are payments received from patients before the actual service is delivered. They can take various forms, such as prepayments for annual check-ups, retainers for specialized medical services, or deposits for surgical procedures. For example, Dr. Smith, who runs a prominent orthopedic clinic, offers a comprehensive wellness package where patients prepay for an entire year's worth of services, including consultations, diagnostics, and follow-up treatments. This prepayment ensures that Dr. Smith has a predictable cash flow to manage his practice's expenses.

Managing advance payments requires a strategic approach to ensure that you meet patient expectations and maintain financial integrity. When patients pay in advance, they're entrusting you with their money based on the promise of future services. Dr. Smith's clinic has developed a robust system to track these prepayments, ensuring that each patient receives the promised services without delay. This system includes automated scheduling, regular reminders, and a dedicated staff member to handle any patient queries related to their prepaid services. By maintaining clear communication and delivering high-quality care consistently, Dr. Smith ensures that his patients are satisfied and likely to renew their packages.

Effective communication is essential in managing advance payments. Patients need to clearly understand what they are paying for, when they will receive the services, and what to expect throughout the process. Dr. Smith's team provides detailed brochures and personalized consultations to explain the wellness package, ensuring that patients are fully informed before making a commitment. This transparency builds trust and enhances patient satisfaction, which is crucial for the long-term success of the advance payment model.

Now, let's talk about the accounting practices for advance payments. When you receive an advance payment, it should be recorded as a liability on your balance sheet. This is because the money hasn't been earned yet; it represents a future obligation to provide services. For instance, if Dr. Smith's clinic receives $10,000 from a patient for a year-long wellness package, this amount is initially recorded as "Deferred Revenue." As the services are provided over the year, portions of this deferred revenue are recognized as earned revenue.

Accurate accounting ensures transparency and prevents financial misstatements. Dr. Smith's accountant records the initial $10,000 as a liability. Each month, as services are rendered, a portion of this amount—say $833.33 per month for 12 months—is moved from deferred revenue to earned revenue. This method provides a clear financial picture, showing both the clinic's obligations and its actual earnings.

Advance payments can significantly impact cash flow by providing immediate liquidity. This influx of cash allows you to invest in your practice, cover operating expenses, and manage unexpected costs without financial strain. Dr. Kim, a pediatrician, offers a prepayment option for annual vaccinations and wellness checks. The advance payments she receives at the beginning of the year allow her to invest in new equipment and technology, enhancing the quality of care she provides. This upfront cash also gives her the financial flexibility to handle any unforeseen expenses without disrupting her practice's operations.

Let's look at some real-world examples to see how effective management of advance payments can benefit your practice. Dr. Patel, who runs a dermatology clinic, offers a skin care subscription service where patients prepay for quarterly treatments and products. By managing these advance payments effectively, Dr. Patel ensures a steady revenue stream throughout the year. Her accountant meticulously records the prepayments as deferred revenue and gradually recognizes them as earned revenue with each treatment session. This practice not only stabilizes cash flow but also allows Dr. Patel to plan for future investments and growth.

Another example is Dr. Martinez, an ophthalmologist, who introduced an advance payment system for LASIK surgeries. Patients pay a deposit upfront, which secures their surgery date and covers pre-operative consultations. This system ensures that Dr. Martinez has the necessary funds to schedule surgeries efficiently and invest in cutting-edge technology. By recording the deposits as liabilities and recognizing them as revenue once the surgeries are performed, Dr. Martinez maintains accurate financial records and ensures compliance with accounting standards.

In conclusion, managing advance payments for future services is a powerful strategy for enhancing your practice's financial stability and growth. By understanding the types of advance payments, implementing effective management strategies, and adopting accurate accounting practices, you can leverage advance payments to create a predictable and steady income stream. Whether it's offering comprehensive wellness packages, prepaid vaccination plans, or subscription services, advance payments provide significant financial benefits. Following the examples of Dr. Smith, Dr. Kim, Dr. Patel, and Dr. Martinez, you can turn advance payments into a strategic advantage for your practice. Let's take control of our financial destiny, master the management of advance payments, and drive our practice toward new heights of success.

CHAPTER 24:

Mastering Income from Joint Ventures

Alright, let's dive deep into an advanced strategy that can catapult your practice's financial health to the next level: income from joint ventures. When you enter into a joint venture or partnership, you're collaborating with other businesses to achieve shared goals. These partnerships can provide a lucrative revenue stream that complements your primary operations. However, managing and accounting for this income requires a strategic approach. We'll explore the intricacies of joint venture income, how to manage these earnings effectively, the necessary accounting practices, and real-world examples to demonstrate the power of successful joint ventures.

First, let's get a clear understanding of what joint venture income is. A joint venture is a business arrangement where two or more parties come together to undertake a specific project or business activity. Each party contributes resources, shares risks, and enjoys the profits. For a medical practice, this might involve partnering with another healthcare provider, a research institution, or even a pharmaceutical company. For instance, Dr. Thompson, who runs a renowned multi-specialty clinic, entered into a joint venture with a leading medical research firm to develop and conduct clinical trials for new treatments. This partnership provided his clinic with a substantial new revenue stream while advancing medical research.

Understanding the nature of joint venture income is crucial. Unlike your primary operational income, which comes directly from patient services, joint venture earnings stem from collaborative projects that leverage the strengths and resources of each partner. This means that while the income can be substantial, it also involves shared control and shared risks. Dr. Thompson's partnership required a clear agreement on how resources would be allocated, how profits would be shared, and how risks would be managed.

Managing joint venture earnings effectively is essential for maximizing the benefits of these partnerships. It starts with establishing clear and detailed agreements that outline the roles, responsibilities, and expectations of each partner. Dr. Thompson's joint venture agreement with the research firm included specifics on how much each party would invest, how the profits would be split, and how decisions would be made. This clarity helped prevent misunderstandings and ensured that both parties were aligned towards common goals.

Effective communication is vital in managing joint ventures. Regular meetings and updates ensure that all partners are on the same page and can address any issues promptly. Dr. Thompson and his partners held monthly meetings to review the progress of their clinical trials, discuss any challenges, and make strategic decisions. These meetings fostered a collaborative environment and kept the project on track.

It's also important to monitor the financial performance of the joint venture closely. This involves tracking expenses, revenues, and profits to ensure that the venture is financially viable. Dr. Thompson's clinic used advanced financial management software to monitor the joint venture's financials in real-time. This allowed them to make informed decisions and adjust their strategies as needed to optimize profitability.

Accounting for joint venture income requires precise and transparent practices. When you receive earnings from a joint venture, it's essential to record them separately from your primary operational income. This distinction helps in providing a clear financial picture and ensures compliance with accounting standards. For example, when Dr. Thompson's clinic received profits from the joint venture, these earnings were recorded under a separate line item called "Joint Venture Income." This categorization distinguished it from revenue generated directly from patient services and maintained the clarity of financial reporting.

The accounting treatment of joint venture income can vary depending on the structure of the venture. In some cases, joint ventures are treated as separate legal entities, and profits are distributed to the partners. In other cases, the venture might be more informal, with each partner recognizing their share of the profits directly. Dr. Thompson's joint venture was structured as a separate legal entity, so his clinic recognized its share of the profits as income from an investment.

Let's dive into some real-world examples to see how effective management of joint venture income can benefit your practice. Dr. Kim, a pediatrician, entered into a joint venture with a local hospital to create a specialized children's health center. This partnership combined Dr. Kim's expertise in pediatric care with the hospital's advanced facilities and resources. The joint venture allowed Dr. Kim to offer a wider range of services to her patients and provided a significant new revenue stream. By maintaining clear agreements and regular communication, the joint venture thrived, benefiting both Dr. Kim's practice and the hospital.

Dr. Lee's dermatology clinic provides another example. She partnered with a pharmaceutical company to conduct clinical trials for new skincare treatments. The joint venture agreement outlined how costs would be shared, how profits would be distributed, and how the trials would be managed. This partnership not only generated substantial income for Dr. Lee's clinic but also enhanced its reputation in the medical community. By meticulously accounting for the joint venture income and maintaining open communication with the pharmaceutical company, Dr. Lee ensured the success and profitability of the venture.

Dr. Martinez, an ophthalmologist, formed a joint venture with a medical device company to develop and test innovative eye care technologies. This partnership leveraged Dr. Martinez's clinical expertise and the company's technological capabilities. The joint venture resulted in significant advancements in eye care and provided a lucrative income stream for Dr. Martinez's clinic. By using advanced financial management tools to monitor the venture's performance and maintaining a clear agreement on profit-sharing and responsibilities, Dr. Martinez maximized the benefits of the joint venture.

Dr. Patel's orthopedic clinic entered into a joint venture with a leading sports medicine research center. This partnership focused on developing new treatments and rehabilitation programs for athletes. The joint venture agreement included detailed terms on investment, profit-sharing, and intellectual property rights. This collaboration not only generated substantial income for Dr. Patel's clinic but also positioned it as a leader in sports medicine. By ensuring accurate accounting practices and maintaining regular communication with the research center, Dr. Patel's clinic reaped significant benefits from the joint venture.

In conclusion, managing and accounting for income from joint ventures is a powerful strategy for enhancing the financial health and growth of your medical practice. By understanding the nature of joint venture income, implementing effective management strategies, and adopting precise accounting practices, you can leverage these partnerships to create significant new revenue streams. Whether it's collaborating with a research firm, partnering with a hospital, or developing new technologies, joint ventures offer substantial financial and professional benefits. Following the examples of Dr. Thompson, Dr. Kim, Dr. Lee, Dr. Martinez, and Dr. Patel, you can turn joint ventures into strategic advantages for your practice. Let's take control of our financial destiny, master the management of joint venture income, and drive our practice toward new heights of success.

CHAPTER 25:

Mastering Special Discounts from Bulk Purchases

Alright, let's talk about a savvy financial move that can save your practice significant money: bulk purchasing agreements. Imagine buying your supplies in larger quantities and getting special discounts that lower your overall costs. This strategy can lead to substantial savings, but these benefits might not be immediately reflected in your cash flow. We're going to explore the benefits of bulk purchasing, how to manage these agreements effectively, the accounting practices you need to adopt, and real-world examples that demonstrate the advantages of this strategy.

First, let's dive into the benefits of bulk purchasing. Buying in bulk allows you to negotiate better prices with suppliers, reducing the cost per unit of the items you need. For instance, Dr. Smith, who runs a bustling dental practice, realized he could save a significant amount by purchasing dental supplies in larger quantities. Instead of buying materials every month, he negotiated a bulk purchasing agreement with his supplier, reducing his costs by 20%. This strategy allowed him to allocate those savings to other critical areas of his practice, such as upgrading equipment and training staff.

Bulk purchasing also ensures that you have a consistent supply of necessary items, reducing the risk of running out of essential materials. This is particularly important in a medical practice, where having the right supplies on hand is crucial for providing uninterrupted patient care. Dr. Smith's bulk purchasing agreement meant that his practice always had a steady supply of gloves, masks, and other disposable items, ensuring smooth operations and consistent patient satisfaction.

Managing bulk purchase agreements requires a strategic approach. It's not just about buying in large quantities; it's about negotiating terms that benefit your practice and maintaining a good relationship with your suppliers. Dr. Smith negotiated terms that included not only a significant discount but also flexible delivery schedules and favorable payment terms. This flexibility allowed him to manage his inventory more effectively, ensuring that his practice wasn't overwhelmed with supplies all at once.

Effective communication with your suppliers is key to managing these agreements. Regularly reviewing the terms and performance of the agreement ensures that both parties are satisfied and that the agreement continues to meet your practice's needs. Dr. Smith's practice held quarterly meetings with their supplier to discuss any issues, review usage patterns, and adjust orders as needed. This proactive approach maintained a positive relationship with the supplier and ensured that the practice continued to receive the best possible terms.

Now, let's talk about the accounting practices for managing special discounts from bulk purchases. When you receive a discount from bulk purchasing, it's important to account for these savings accurately. Initially, the total expenditure might appear higher because you're buying in larger quantities, but the per-unit cost is lower, and the overall savings can be significant over time.

For example, Dr. Smith's accountant recorded the bulk purchase at the total amount paid but noted the per-unit cost reduction as a separate line item in the accounting records. This approach provided a clear picture of the actual cost savings achieved through the bulk purchase agreement. The practice also kept track of inventory levels to ensure that the supplies were used efficiently and didn't go to waste.

The impact of bulk purchasing on cash flow can be substantial. While the initial outlay might be higher, the long-term savings can free up cash that can be invested back into the practice. Dr. Kim, a pediatrician, implemented a bulk purchasing strategy for vaccines and medical supplies. The upfront cost was higher, but the significant savings allowed her to invest in new diagnostic equipment and expand her clinic's services. Over time, the reduced costs contributed to improved cash flow and greater financial stability for her practice.

Let's explore some real-world examples to see how effective management of bulk purchasing agreements can benefit your practice. Dr. Patel, who runs a dermatology clinic, partnered with a supplier to purchase skincare products in bulk. By negotiating a favorable bulk purchasing agreement, she reduced her costs by 25%. These savings allowed her to offer competitive pricing to her patients, attracting more clients and increasing her overall revenue. Dr. Patel's accountant meticulously tracked the cost savings and ensured that the financial statements reflected the reduced expenditure, providing a clear picture of the practice's financial health.

Another example is Dr. Martinez, an ophthalmologist, who needed to purchase expensive surgical supplies. By entering into a bulk purchasing agreement with a supplier, he was able to secure a substantial discount. The initial cost was high, but the long-term savings allowed him to invest in state-of-the-art surgical equipment, enhancing the quality of care he provided. Dr. Martinez's practice carefully tracked the inventory and accounted for the special discounts, ensuring accurate financial reporting and strategic reinvestment of the savings.

In conclusion, managing and accounting for special discounts from bulk purchases is a powerful strategy for enhancing the financial health and stability of your medical practice. By understanding the benefits of bulk purchasing, implementing effective management strategies, and adopting precise accounting practices, you can leverage these discounts to create significant cost savings. Whether it's purchasing dental supplies, skincare products, vaccines, or surgical supplies, bulk purchasing agreements offer substantial financial advantages. Following the examples of Dr. Smith, Dr. Kim, Dr. Patel, and Dr. Martinez, you can turn bulk purchasing into a strategic advantage for your practice. Let's take control of our financial destiny, master the management of bulk purchases, and drive our practice toward new heights of success.

CONCLUSION:

Unleashing Hidden Cash Flow in Your Medical Practice

Alright, let's wrap this up with a powerful message about transforming your medical practice's financial landscape. Throughout this book, we've delved into various financial strategies that can help you uncover and manage hidden cash flow in your practice. It's not just about keeping the lights on; it's about driving growth, ensuring sustainability, and maximizing the potential of every dollar that flows through your doors. By leveraging the insights and strategies discussed here, you can take your practice to new heights of financial success.

Effectively managing hidden cash flow requires more than just a basic understanding of your finances. It demands a deep dive into the financial mechanisms at play, an acute awareness of where your money is coming from and going, and the savvy to optimize every aspect of your financial operations. Whether it's mastering deferred revenue, capitalizing on bulk purchase discounts, or tapping into the lucrative potential of joint ventures, each strategy is a tool in your arsenal to enhance financial planning, ensure transparency, and maintain the financial health of your practice.

Consider Dr. Thompson, who implemented a comprehensive approach to managing deferred revenue from subscription services. By recording and recognizing revenue accurately, he not only ensured compliance but also gained a clear picture of his practice's financial health. This clarity allowed him to make informed decisions about investing in new technologies and expanding his services. Dr. Thompson didn't just keep his practice afloat; he propelled it forward, leveraging financial insight to drive growth.

Then there's Dr. Lee, who took advantage of vendor financing arrangements to upgrade her clinic without draining her cash reserves. By negotiating favorable terms and maintaining rigorous accounting practices, she kept her cash flow steady and her practice equipped with the latest technology. Dr. Lee's story is a testament to the power of strategic financial management—showing that with the right approach, you can achieve stability and growth simultaneously.

Dr. Kim's experience with bulk purchasing agreements highlights another crucial aspect of financial mastery. By negotiating significant discounts on essential supplies, she reduced her operating costs and freed up capital for critical investments. This proactive approach not only improved her practice's profitability but also ensured that she could continue providing top-notch care without financial strain.

And let's not forget Dr. Patel, who expertly managed advance payments for future services. By setting up clear, transparent accounting practices and maintaining strong communication with her patients, she turned prepayments into a reliable source of cash flow. This strategy provided her with the financial flexibility to navigate unexpected expenses and invest in her practice's future.

Each of these examples underscores a fundamental truth: effectively managing hidden cash flow is about more than just keeping track of dollars and cents. It's about understanding the financial ecosystem of your practice and using that knowledge to make strategic decisions. It's about being proactive, not reactive; strategic, not opportunistic. And most importantly, it's about seeing beyond the immediate balance sheet to the long-term health and success of your practice.

To get started on this transformative journey, take a moment to assess where you stand. Scan the QR code below to discover just how much hidden cash flow you might be giving away every month. This isn't just a number; it's an opportunity—a chance to take control, maximize your revenue, and elevate your practice to the next level.

Imagine a future where every financial decision is backed by solid data, where your practice is not just surviving but thriving. Picture the freedom to invest in new technologies, expand your services, and provide the best possible care to your patients, all without the constant worry of cash flow issues. That future starts now, with the strategies and insights you've gained from this book.

So, don't let another dollar slip through your fingers. Embrace the journey of discovering and managing hidden cash flow in your medical practice. Take the first step today, and let's get started on a path to unparalleled financial success. Your practice deserves it, your patients deserve it, and you deserve it. Welcome to the future of financially empowered medical practice management. Let's make it happen!

To get started, scan the QR code below to find out just how much hidden cash flow you're giving away every month. Don't let another dollar slip through your fingers. It's time to take control, maximize your revenue, and elevate your practice to the next level. Welcome to the journey of discovering hidden cash flow in your medical practice. Let's get started!

www.ingramcontent.com/pod-product-compliance
Lightning Source LLC
Chambersburg PA
CBHW071831210526
45479CB00001B/91